5 Steps to Building Resilience in Today's Fast-Paced & Uncertain World

Conquering Work Stress, Gaining Confidence, Relationship Hurdles, Financial Struggles, Personal, Professional Growth, and Bouncing Back From Setbacks

Jed Lindsay

© Copyright 2024 - All rights reserved.

The content contained within this book may not be reproduced, duplicated or transmitted without direct written permission from the author or the publisher.

Under no circumstances will any blame or legal responsibility be held against the publisher, or author, for any damages, reparation, or monetary loss due to the information contained within this book, either directly or indirectly.

Legal Notice:

This book is copyright protected. It is only for personal use. You cannot amend, distribute, sell, use, quote or paraphrase any part, or the content within this book, without the consent of the author or publisher.

Disclaimer Notice:

Please note the information contained within this document is for educational and entertainment purposes only. All effort has been executed to present accurate, up to date, reliable, complete information. No warranties of any kind are declared or implied. Readers acknowledge that the author is not engaged in the rendering of legal, financial, medical or professional advice. The content within this book has been derived from various sources. Please consult a licensed professional before attempting any techniques outlined in this book.

By reading this document, the reader agrees that under no circumstances is the author responsible for any losses, direct or indirect, that are incurred as a result of the use of the information contained within this document, including, but not limited to, errors, omissions, or inaccuracies.

Table of Contents

INTRODUCTION 1

PART 1: THE BASICS OF RESILIENCE 9

   CHAPTER 1: THE RESILIENCE BLUEPRINT—UNRAVELING THE MYSTERY OF ENDURANCE 11
      The Concept of Resilience 13
      Resilient Rarities 17
      The Resilience Ripple 26
      Resilience Realities and Myths... 30
   CHAPTER 2: THE BIOLOGY OF BOUNCING BACK—HOW OUR BODIES FOSTER RESILIENCE .. 33
      The Resilience Matrix: The Brain-Body Connection in Resilience................ 35
      The Role of Genetics in Resilience.. 37
      Neurobiology of Resilience 39
      Environmental Influences on Resilience Development 41
      Decoding the Neural Mechanisms Behind Stress Adaptation and Resilience 43

PART 2: REBOUNDING MENTALLY AND EMOTIONALLY 47

   CHAPTER 3: RISING ABOVE—TURNING LIFE'S CHALLENGES INTO STEPPING STONES.......... 49
      Challenges that Test Resilience: Identifying Life's Common Adversities...... 51
      Overcoming Life's Common Adversities.. 53
      Personal Stories of Overcoming Adversity 56
      Learning from Adversity 58
   CHAPTER 4: THE ART OF THE COMEBACK—OVERCOMING SETBACKS AND EMBRACING FAILURE... 63
      Confronting Setbacks and Failures 64
      Turning Setbacks into Opportunities 66
      Bounce Back Better: Techniques and Mindsets for Rising Above Failure 69
   CHAPTER 5: THE POWER OF THE MIND—CULTIVATING MENTAL FORTITUDE FOR RESILIENCE 73
      Mental Might and Resilience 74
      Strategies for Cultivating Mental Strength.. 78
      Mind Over Matter... 81

PART 3: AMPLIFYING RESILIENCE THROUGH SOCIAL BONDS AND POSITIVE HABITS 85

   CHAPTER 6: THE CIRCLE OF STRENGTH—HARNESSING SOCIAL SUPPORT IN BUILDING RESILIENCE... 87

The Power of We: Social Connections in Resilience Building 89
Nurturing Bonds 92
The Role of Communication in Relationships 95
Strategies for Effective Communication and Seeking Help............ 98
CHAPTER 7: DAILY DOSES OF RESILIENCE—HABITS THAT BOLSTER YOUR BOUNCE-BACK ABILITY 103
Habits of Steel... 105
Self-Care: Your Path to Personal Wellness 108
Self-Care Tips 110
Beat the Burnout: Effective Strategies for Stress Management..... 114
Busting Stress and Burnout Myths 118
Practical Strategies for Managing Stress and Preventing Burnout 121

PART 4: VITAL TACTICS FOR FOSTERING RESILIENCE IN OTHERS AND AT WORK 125

CHAPTER 8: GROWING GRIT—NURTURING RESILIENCE IN TOMORROW'S LEADERS.......... 127
Shaping Resilience: The Crucial Role of Parents, Educators, and Caregivers 129
Understanding Resilience in Different Age Groups......................134
Growing Strong: Strategies for Boosting Resilience in Youth 136
The Power of Fostering Healthy Physical Coping......................... 139
The Power of Fostering Healthy Emotional Coping 140
CHAPTER 9: THRIVING AMID TURBULENCE—BUILDING RESILIENCE IN THE WORKPLACE ... 143
Workplace Resilience: A Key to Professional Triumph................. 144
Unmasking Common Challenges and Stressors........................... 146
The Impact of Workplace Stressors 149
Strategies for Boosting Resilience and Balancing Professional Life........... 154

PART 5: ENDURANCE AND LONGEVITY IN RESILIENCE 159

CHAPTER 10: EMOTIONAL ARMOR—BUILDING RESILIENCE FROM THE INSIDE OUT.......... 161
The Role of Emotional Intelligence in Building Resilience........... 161
Emotional Mastery 165
Path to Positivity.. 175
CHAPTER 11: STAND STRONG IN THE STORM—ENHANCING RESILIENCE IN TIMES OF CRISIS 181
Understanding Crisis Challenges and Emergencies 182
Resilience Guidance for Stressful Times....................................... 184
Identifying Emotions During Crises 187
Managing Emotions During Crises 191
CHAPTER 12: THE LONG GAME—SUSTAINING RESILIENCE FOR LIFELONG WELL-BEING 195
Perseverance Prevails: The Importance of Ongoing Resilience Nurturing..199
Building Resilience Practices.. 202
Reflection, Gratitude, Compassion—The Trio of Sustained Resilience 205

CONCLUSION 209

GLOSSARY 211

REFERENCES 215

Acknowledgment and Dedication

To my beloved mother Jane and my two superheroes, Elijah and Eden Thoms, who have been my unwavering rock of support and love, I humbly dedicate this tribute to your steadfast strength, endless compassion, and boundless love that you bring to my life. Your presence fills my days with joy. You have been the guiding lights in my life, the pillars of strength that hold me up through every storm. Your love, wisdom, and unwavering support have shaped me into who I am today. I am eternally grateful for your presence in my life and the love you show me. Thank you for being my constants, cheerleaders, and greatest blessings. This dedication is for you, my precious family, who mean more to me than words can express.

I want to express my profound appreciation to everyone who worked tirelessly to make this book a reality. Your commitment and unwavering support have been invaluable. I would particularly like to acknowledge those who have been a source of hope during my most challenging times: Ayo Obe, Cadainne Hart, Kelis Richard, Rita Sterling, Olivia Busagwa, Geraldine Oyela, Auntie Harriet, Candida Netto, Susan Abboh, Fauzia, Elizabeth, and Erich. I want to give special thanks to Precious, whose reminders of the power of resilience inspired me every day. Your encouragement kept me going when I felt I could no longer continue. To Vuzi and family, your limitless love and support have meant everything to me. Thank you all from the bottom of my heart.

My dear reader, I am truly grateful to you for purchasing my book! Your support means everything to me, and I am deeply honored by your interest in my work. I hope you find the book insightful and enjoyable, and I appreciate any feedback you may have. Your support as a reader is invaluable to me, and I cannot thank you enough for choosing to explore the pages of my book.

Introduction

Many of us are struggling more than ever these days to bounce back from difficult situations. Recent research shows as many as one in four adults worldwide, including even healthcare workers, experience low resilience (Janitra et al., 2023). This inability to withstand challenges profoundly affects our well-being. When we're in such a weakened state, our mental health suffers, relationships become strained, career progress stagnates, and overall happiness decreases. Without the skills to recover from hardship, life becomes so much more painful to navigate. If left unaddressed, this state risks destroying countless people's potential and quality of life over the long run. Building resilience is vitally important for protecting against these serious outcomes. We must prioritize cultivating ways to withstand adversity so we can thrive regardless of whatever obstacles come our way in the future.

Having resilience means you have the mental fortitude and viewpoint (through various strategies) to recover from tough situations in life, like failures, tragic events, or things not working out as you planned. When something knocks them down, resilient people don't get stuck there; they refuse to let current problems stop them from pursuing their goals.

Resilient people make a conscious effort to strengthen their emotional skills, ones that help them rise above circumstances beyond their control. These circumstances are often the things that get in the way of people bettering themselves or advancing in their careers. Resilient people know that developing grit, optimism, and the ability to adapt is so important for overcoming obstacles and keeping progress on track, even when faced with hardship. Building these inner strengths provides more control over your attitude and power over your actions, so outside storms rolling through can't keep you down for good.

Having resilience can protect us from getting stuck in negative mindsets when tough times roll around. It's important to remember that difficulties and failures are a part of everyone's life. However, instead of falling apart after these setbacks, resilient people transform failures into opportunities to learn and better themselves. They don't let difficult emotions like fear, embarrassment, or regret hold them back from continuing to develop. Resilient people still acknowledge they're not perfect, and show themselves kindness instead of harsh criticism. They also cultivate supportive relationships, routines, and strategies that keep their inner drive alive despite temporary defeats. This way, resilient individuals don't let fleeting problems ruin their long-term happiness, motivation, or chances for an even brighter future. Developing inner strength and an attitude of growth over fragility can help you ride out life's ups and downs.

When life gets demanding, resilience makes all the difference. There are the everyday stresses that we mentioned, but life's demands show up in many other ways as well. Relationships can also take their toll through breakups, arguments, and disappointments. Then there'll be challenges to our health and other tough changes in routine or family dynamics that we'll all face. Without the skills to cope, some people understandably drown in their problems or turn to unhealthy ways to cope just to escape feeling overwhelmed. But having lifelong resilience means understanding that hard times are inevitable, and having the strength inside to not only withstand them, but to grow stronger from them. Resilience protects against being crushed under challenges, and instead powers our ability to survive and even be renewed by life's difficulties. It's a protective quality we'd all benefit from cultivating.

Why waste time feeling anxious and worn down when you can start building up your resilience today? This book lays out a powerful yet simple method known as B.R.A.V.E. B.R.A.V.E. is a handy framework for boosting your inner strength to face anything life throws at you. It lets you overcome worries about not having it all figured out by strengthening the core abilities we all possess deep down. You'll learn how small changes can lead to big results. So, why continue to be dragged down by worries, fear, and fatigue? Take control right now through the resilience strategies in these pages.

Developing resilience is key to feeling truly content and in control at all times, not just when things are good externally. It gives you more power over your own well-being rather than leaving it up to outside forces you can't control. Resilience helps you focus on playing to your strengths even when faced with challenges, instead of getting stuck in our insecurities.

The strategies in this guide can help you strengthen your inner resources to better withstand difficulties, the type that even successful people and strong relationships struggle with from time to time. Don't let temporary setbacks ruin your view of life overall; use them as chances to grow. Heal by working through the five steps of the B.R.A.V.E. method below:

- **B for basics of resilience**: Before attempting to adopt resilient mindsets in daily situations, first grasp the theories that empower individuals to frame struggles through hopeful lenses rather than victim mentalities.

- **R for rebounding mentally and emotionally**: Adapt using coping mechanisms, allowing for flexibility when confronting unmet expectations head-on. Develop skills for exhibiting grace under pressure, regardless of circumstances.

- **A for amplifying resilience through social bonds and positive habits**: We sustain resilience by proactively surrounding ourselves with supportive people while developing routines, rest, and self-care habits to prevent burnout.

- **V for vital tactics for fostering resilience in others and at work**: Beyond the personal sphere, learn ways of cultivating resilient cultures across families, teams, and organizations overloaded by evolving workplace demands.

- **E for endurance and longevity in resilience**: Explore evergreen principles and advanced techniques to prevent resilience plateauing, but rather continuing growth across life's seasons.

By taking the time to learn and apply the five key parts of this resilience model, you'll significantly strengthen your ability to withstand setbacks without getting worn down. Instead of roadblocks impeding progress, you'll see hardships as chances to show grit and spread optimism where others may give up. Mastering the B.R.A.V.E. method unlocks lasting strategies for facing life's difficulties from a position of strength, hope, and growth rather than fragility. When you commit to building up these inner resources, you gain power over whether outside forces will truly derail your journey or just make you even tougher. This guide holds the keys—are you ready to level up your resilience?

We could all use more everyday heroes—people who can face storms with optimism instead of feeling like a hopeless victim or just giving up Now's the chance to call on your inner hero and start gradually building up your resilience for whatever challenges come your way. You never know what's around the corner, so fill your toolbox with mental strategies to tap into no matter what obstacles arise in your health, relationships, or career journey. Building these stores of inner fortitude takes brave work, but it means that when uncertainty strikes next, you'll be as prepared as possible to hold your head high. Your future self will be grateful you made the choice today to start cultivating resilience skills.

Commit to building resilience competencies, not just short-term 'life hacks,' by incrementally applying this book's comprehensive, science-backed frameworks. Grow substantially from learning how to:

- **Understand resilience in-depth**: Gain insight into what builds inner strength to face hard times. Learn strategies centered on empowering mindsets rather than feeling helpless.

- **Boost your mental edge**: Handle work stresses, financial swings, health issues, or relationship troubles better by facing fears head-on instead of being overwhelmed. Turn your anxiety into action.

- **Level up your problem-solving**: Deal with dilemmas and hurdles through creative solutions rather than feeling like a victim which only makes things worse. When issues come, you'll be ready to handle them in a solution-focused way rather than feeling doomed.

- **Manage your emotions effectively**: Learn healthy ways to deal with feeling let down, sad, annoyed, or resentful without getting consumed by depression or feeling stuck. Make progress by truly experiencing and processing your emotions without letting anything destroy you emotionally.

- **Believe in yourself more**: Silencing negative thoughts and battling perceptions of low self-worth is key. Doubting yourself can hold you back from opportunities. Tap into your fullest abilities by realizing your strength comes from within, not needing approval from others.

- **Build resilience through habits and support**: Develop routines, surround yourself with positive environments, and nurture relationships that reinforce your ability to withstand hardship. Make yourself confident when faced with challenges instead of fragile by strengthening your resilience over time.

- **Skills you can share with others**: Resilience building isn't just for yourself, but can also help improve teams, families, and other groups facing big problems requiring shared perseverance. Learn approaches for fostering strength-based attitudes in these groups facing situations of cross-stress that risk individual or collective well-being.

- **Sustainable growth trajectory**: You'll expand your resilience more and more over a lifetime of growth and failures. View setbacks as opportunities and gain perspective on what went wrong, instead of losses defining your future. Crises don't have to control you when you can power through them and keep growing.

As you learn from each chapter, use the B.R.A.V.E. method right away to help you through tough times. By staying strong and flexible, you'll come out on the other side having grown even stronger. Finish this book knowing you can get through anything once you leave past negativity and hurt behind and realize your potential. Your best days are ahead of you. Why? Because you've faced difficult situations bravely and become wiser already. You've got this: with perseverance and heart, you'll live fully and happily. Keep learning, keep shining—you've got so much wonderful life still ahead of you!

Before we dive into building grit for the long haul, let me give you some backstory so you know I've been deep in the trenches too. I haven't arrived here easily, preaching from some pedestal on high. Resilience entered my life the hard way after nearly losing everything worth living for.

Several years ago, I free fell into a pit blacker than night and couldn't find any light. My fiancé, whom I thought I'd grow old with, left suddenly. And not just left—I caught him sleeping with my best friend, who knew she was stabbing a knife in my back. Believe it or not, this situation only got worse. I found out just before having our baby boy, whom I birthed in tears rather than joy. Those days bled together into nothing, my mind constantly in survival mode. My newborn was attached to my breast seemingly every hour as I choked back sobs, To put it bluntly, I was drowning in grief.

Yeah, no one dreams of single motherhood overnight, struggling to wash cloth diapers because there is no energy for laundry. I starved, exhausted by screaming fits from my child. My torn-up body recoiled at his grasping hands. Resentment poisoned that precious baby bond every hallmark card celebrates. Where were those fireworks of love the instant our eyes met?

The hormone crash post-birth brought dark clouds to my mind too. Heavy thoughts pointed to "easy outs" to eternally silence the engulfing pain. I sank under waves of despair so black and so numb that I started rationalizing some warped logic around breaking free.

But just when I considered catching the train to nowhere, a knowing beyond words sparked inside, declaring, "Not today, girl." Call it brain wiring, angel whispers, destiny—whatever it was shook me awake. If not for my boy, who still needed his mama to make it somehow, I might have laid down defeated right there, even with life stretched long ahead.

Yet that flicker of shifting internal priority birthed a turning point. I called out for help. While pride dies hard, I confess to being less all right than the cheery mask I put on conveyed. Doctors adjusted medications, clearing brain fog plaguing basic tasks like eating or bathing. A counselor ministered healing truth to my battered identity with equal parts gentle grace and bold conviction.

Little by little, choice by choice, I rose, resurgent with new eyes on this radically altered landscape. By acknowledging vulnerability in a safe community, my voice returned, and resiliency emerged—weak initially but gathering strength daily. Where death once tempted, I now saw dreams newly awakened. I learned to mother my baby boy with humor and delight as he showed off new tricks like rolling over that I nearly missed. My heart thawed toward his precious being, so innocent and naive of his rough entrance. I took the first steps toward recovering the self-confidence that was ravaged by cruel betrayal.

Resilience planted seeds in the ashes to bloom hope anew. I write this survival story now to assure you too—if you too are trapped under piles of stress, unable to visualize clearing the rubble that is suffocating your dreams—that courage comes with each rising sun. Others who overcame stand ready to grip your hand when strength fails, to fan embers subsiding inside until you reignite the fire of resilience again. We go through this together, friend. Where you see no way forward, it awaits nearby, through another's sight lifted higher. Let me lift you the way others have compassionately lifted me. The worst darkness still gives way to light somehow, some way, beyond what we can see.

So, take my hand, weary one, finding insufficient strength to take the next steps obscured ahead. Allow me to steady your shoulders so you stand tall again when it feels impossible to stand alone. We will venture ahead together until joy's first faint rays pierce the darkness once more; after this long, bitterest night passes into day. A new dawn comes, for certain. Follow my words now to find how resilience may rise steadily in every soul, even if it senses that the worst still lies ahead. If we fall, we will fall forward into growth, awaiting our willingness to continue onwards.

Part 1:
The Basics of Resilience

Chapter 1:
The Resilience Blueprint—Unraveling the Mystery of Endurance

It's natural for tough times to come up, such as problems at work, money troubles, difficulties with family, or health issues. It seems like the media always warns about some new worry to concern ourselves with as well! It's no wonder many people feel stressed. Sometimes sharing concerns with others brings short-term comfort by making us feel less alone. But what matters most is what we *do*, not just saying how things make us feel. While talking through issues has its place, taking positive steps, however small, is what eventually leads to solutions and growth instead of lingering in unease. We've all got the ability within us to rise, no matter what obstacles come our way.

In this chapter, the first pitstop in our shared resilience journey, you'll gain mental fortitude to help you navigate rough patches. You'll learn how to navigate problems with confidence and optimism, even when it's tough to see clearly through periods of worry, sadness, or negativity. Arming yourself with these tools early means you'll be all set to take on challenges in stride whenever tough times roll around.

We all need to retire the myth that some personalities are naturally weaker while others are naturally tougher when facing hardships like loss or uncertainty. The truth is that our brains are made for adaptability, not predetermined weaknesses. The real game-changer? Retooling our instincts so problems provoke our strength, not defeat. When life gets tough, aim to react in ways that strengthen, not weaken, your resolve. No one should be a victim to circumstances beyond their control, because everyone can develop resilience! You've got untapped inner grit just waiting to be uncovered.

As you continue along your path, expect that there will be obstacles in your way. How you view each situation, whether as an opportunity or a roadblock, is up to your perspective. To start strengthening your resilience, two important ideas to familiarize yourself with are locus of control, and fixed vs. growth mindsets. Locus of control refers to whether you see outside forces or your efforts as what determines your outcomes, while mindset shapes how you respond when things don't go your way. With a growth mindset, you see challenges as things you can learn from rather than things that prove you're incapable. Grasping these core frameworks will give you strong foundations for navigating unpredictability with flexibility, optimism, and self-belief.

When facing challenges, it's easy to fall into faulty patterns of thinking that don't serve us well.

- We blame others or outside forces for how we feel internally, instead of taking responsibility for our emotional responses.

- We get paralyzed by new experiences instead of meeting them with open-minded curiosity.

- We spiral into worst-case scenario thinking, assuming the worst possible outcome is guaranteed rather than recognizing that every situation holds multiple possible outcomes, good and bad.

Moving past these limited perceptions is important for our ability to stay optimistic and resilient through life's ups and downs. We would do well to reflect on where our thoughts may be flawed, let go of external attributions, practice embracing the unknown, and catch ourselves when spiraling into depression or negative thinking. We adopt all of these strategies so that we can approach each experience, however difficult, with greater clarity and flexibility.

After learning the core principles of true resilience, we are better equipped to avoid common traps that undermine people.

One myth is that smooth sailing through life is the default, rather than ups and downs being a natural part of life. This invincibility myth leads to outrage and anger when hardship strikes. However, suffering is woven into the human experience. While hard times may feel unfair, meeting difficulties with calmness and compassion for oneself and others is better for the soul. Becoming fired up changes nothing, but keeping calm and showing empathy can ease the pain for all involved. Grounding ourselves, in reality, helps maintain perspective when storms arrive; they do not negate our worth or strength but are opportunities to demonstrate grace.

Some take on far more than they can handle alone, to the point of burning out, and then feel the world has let them down rather than accepting their limits. We ease unnecessary strain by acknowledging where and when we need help from others, instead of trying to do it all independently.

Others get stuck reliving past pains, passively waiting for circumstances to change rather than driving their growth. But transformations start from the inside out, not from the outside in. Our situations are either problems or possibilities, depending on our frame of mind. Rather than seeing ourselves as helpless victims of fate, we can view challenges as opportunities and take empowered action over our lives from a place of strength and agency. Interdependence and inner drive are both important parts of the resilience equation.

Feelings of grief or despair after traumatic events are valid, and it's important to process them. This is where getting help can prove a wise decision, perhaps from loved ones. Their support can ease suffering when moving past hard times feels impossible alone. However, blaming others or larger societal problems doesn't empower us or enable healing; taking charge of our own lives is what builds power within.

Resilience isn't a passive thing; it's an active choice strengthened through cultivating new habits of thought, even when the future feels uncertain. Our biology and upbringing shape us significantly, but each person ultimately grows to withstand challenges by reframing fearful reactions and beliefs into anchors of stability. Facing whatever hardships come tomorrow with determination rather than weakness of spirit depends on this inner work. We all have the capacity to transform vulnerability into strength.

The Concept of Resilience

Resilience, our ability to withstand difficulties and use challenges as opportunities to grow, is so important for people and societies dealing with today's rapidly changing world. Resilience is about more than just getting through hard times; it allows us to emerge stronger with more wisdom and compassion. Facing shared hardships together with a spirit of resilience promotes human connection. Exploring the deeper aspects of what resilience means can serve as a useful guide for fully developing these vital inner resources. Mastering resilience skills provides a foundation for navigating life's uncertainties with purpose, empathy, and empowerment.

In essence, resilience means having the strength to bounce back after extremely difficult life changes and challenges that alter who you are. Like how some flowers manage to thrive in harsh environments, resilient people face hardships with perseverance and a drive to better themselves. Through resilience, we transform suffering into personal development and wisdom. While some resilience may come naturally, it is also a skill that can be developed over a lifetime (Chan, 2021). The choices we make, our daily routines, and the relationships that support us all shape how we view and respond to obstacles. Resilience grows as we learn to approach tests and trials as opportunities rather than burdens, with flexibility instead of rigidity. Staying close to others through tough times also reinforces our ability to weather storms and grow stronger because of them.

It's important to understand how resilience differs from just having determination. While grit keeps people pushing toward their goals no matter what, that alone isn't sustainable and can take a mental or physical toll without balance. Resilience is about grit mixed with flexibility—knowing when you need to take a new approach rather than hitting your head against a brick wall. A resilient mindset means paying attention to what's possible and accepting changes and limitations in yourself and situations over time. It's about being willing to adapt your path to fulfillment instead of rigidly insisting on one strategy that isn't working. Resilience acknowledges realities while still pursuing your dreams. Where grit keeps charging no matter what, resilience incorporates periodic shifts and self-care to reach your destination no matter what road you take towards it.

Unlike simple optimism, which means hoping things will get better on their own, resilience requires actively facing difficult emotions head-on. When tough times come, being resilient means choosing to not get overwhelmed by negative thoughts that nothing can get better. Instead of avoiding pain, resilience means leaning bravely into discomfort and looking for any lessons that can come out of the situation. It's about finding small victories that can help you keep moving forward, even when major setbacks happen. Rather than just waiting for motivation to return on its own, resilience is rolling up your sleeves and consciously working to find purpose or positive opportunities for change within the challenges.

Types of Resilience

Four interdependent dimensions of resilience support the full actualization of potential:

1. **Physical resilience**: Working on your overall health, fitness, and nutrition makes your body better equipped to handle challenges like illness, injury, or stressful life changes as you go through them. As time goes by, staying active can protect your independence by preventing or reducing issues related to aging. Making exercise a regular part of each day also helps keep your mobility, joints, and energy levels high. Taking good care of your physical self, in general, means you'll be better able to weather tough times without suffering negative health effects. When difficulties come up, having established healthy lifestyle habits will help fortify your body against potential breakdowns.

2. **Mental resilience**: Working intentionally to reinforce the connections in our brains allows us to gain wisdom from what we go through. As we practice looking at situations from new perspectives, we get better at adapting when facing unfamiliar or challenging situations. Mentally resilient people are open to new experiences, even during unsettled times, instead of holding on tightly to one narrow view of things. They approach strong emotions with a focus on learning and improving. Over the years, knowledge builds up as resilient thinking becomes a habit; each experience transforms how we think rather than getting stuck in our rigid patterns. This flexible mental approach is stronger for weathering life's ups and downs.

3. **Emotional resilience**: Handling feelings in a healthy, constructive way makes it easier to roll with life's punches. Dealing with difficult changes doesn't have to derail you when you can skillfully process your emotions. This comes from genuinely acknowledging hard times for yourself and others, rather than ignoring hard feelings. Facing emotions head-on with validation, without judgment, helps make turbulence feel normal and manageable. Resilient people can experience intense reactions without being controlled by them, instead channeling that energy into healthy outlets. By understanding emotional cycles, intense feelings don't have to lead down an unproductive or destructive path.

4. **Social resilience**: It's easier to face challenges when you don't have to do it alone. Being around supportive people who lift your mood, take care of themselves, and see the bright side of challenges acts as an optimistic life raft when times get rough. Friends, family, coworkers, and community keep you from getting pulled under by isolation when problems feel overwhelming. Receiving feedback with compassion instead of criticism from people who've also struggled prevents drowning and drives further growth. Individual resilience is multiplied when gained through relationships where struggles are shared, ensuring that everyone involved gains strength together over time.

Resilience is never a fixed state; it develops gradually through experience facing challenges over time. Be patient with yourself, as these skills take time to build. While difficulties may feel overwhelming now, commit to viewing struggles as opportunities to strengthen your abilities to adapt and endure, whatever uncertainty lies ahead. While it may not feel like immense progress is being made at first, consciously putting yourself through the process will eventually compound that learning. In time, through building your resilience, you will then have the tools and wisdom to help others through their hardships too. With patience, each problem overcome can help make you better equipped to withstand whatever life may bring.

Psychological Roots of Resilience

These days, resilience is a commonly discussed goal as societies aim to prepare people for constant change. However, scientific research on resilience through the field of psychology started growing much later than the initial focus in medicine on diagnosing mental health issues (Fleming and Ledogar, 2018). In the early years of psychiatry, especially after the traumatic effects of World Wars I and II, the dominant approach was discovering and labeling mental illnesses. There was little to no focus on promoting mental wellness for those without problems. Over time, the focus has shifted more toward understanding what allows some people to adapt and even thrive amid difficulties, rather than just treating dysfunctions. Now resilience is at the forefront as we learn more about cultivating strengths instead of solely fixing weaknesses.

Resilient Rarities

While everyone's resilience may fluctuate depending on the situation, there are some consistent qualities in people who tend to bounce back well when times get tough. Learning about these common characteristics, attitudes, and actions that set steadily resilient folks apart can be insightful. It allows you to strengthen your ability to roll with life's ups and downs and intentionally build up those strengths proactively. Facing challenges is inevitable, so gaining insight into resilience traits empowers you to better prepare your mindset and reactions internally, rather than just hoping to withstand whatever obstacles come your way down the line. The more you understand what builds fortitude in others, the better equipped you'll feel to meet personal storms head-on in the future.

By recognizing the attitudes that allow people to sustain achievement through rocky times, we can spark our abilities to withstand life's inevitable challenges and changes. Not with arrogance, but with compassion for our shared vulnerability. All of us will face obstacles, but by studying how resilience works, we gain insight into fortifying our approach. It's about embracing both strengths and weaknesses, so the inevitable hurdles ahead don't mean the end but rather a chance to rise.

Self-Awareness

We all have inner strengths we can tap into when challenging times strike. Cultivating self-awareness is key; it's about taking quiet moments to reflect on both your natural talents and areas where you need support. Those who gracefully weather life's storms tend to have real clarity on who they are deep down, including what they bring to the table and where they require compassion. This grounded sense of self isn't built overnight but instead develops over a lifetime of moments spent building self-understanding. With awareness comes the power to remember what matters, even when sadness or fear tries to shake your center.

Everyone has areas where, when under pressure, they tend to react in ways that don't serve them well. Self-aware people recognize their vulnerabilities, like withdrawing from difficult emotions or being too sensitive to feedback. At the same time, they work proactively on healthier strategies, such as seeking support from caring people who offer honest perspectives in a kind spirit. They also respect what recharges their batteries, such as quiet time if they're more introverted, especially when outer expectations risk draining them completely. The resilient path is about not only honoring our natural edges, but deliberately cultivating empowering attitudes, relationships, and habits proven to nourish well-being even during life's toughest patches. With self-insight and determination, we can overcome unhealthy patterns and build the inner strength to face any challenges that come our way.

Being self-aware means not just recognizing your natural strengths but also spots that need work so you can handle life's difficulties with flexibility. Resilient people consciously craft lives that align with who they truly are at their core and leverage their strengths, rather than stressing about what others expect of them. They understand success isn't defined by titles or comparisons, so their self-worth isn't dependent on external factors alone. This anchored sense of self allows bumps in the road to hurt less when desirable outcomes change unexpectedly.

By focusing on natural abilities and continuing personal growth at your own pace, you develop the confidence and security to roll with life's punches instead of crumbling under them. Build from the inside out, and your resilience will be ready to carry you through whatever challenges may come.

Self-Control

Research clearly shows resilience is a strength we can consciously build up, much like athletes train their bodies (Yang et al., 2019). Studies found people skilled at bouncing back during hard times pause and examine their reactions rather than acting on initial fears or frustration. This brief delay allows them to respond thoughtfully rather than desperately.

Do you know the famous marshmallow test? Kids who are better able to delay eating one treat for the promise of a bigger reward given later on generally achieve more than adults. They had stronger willpower to pause their urges and think ahead (Saxler et al., 2016). Resilient people act similarly when pushed. With practice, we overcome our automatic reactions and empower the logical parts of our minds to steer us during difficulties. By developing mental discipline, our instincts grow to forge ahead no matter what obstacles we hit. We've trained our minds like muscles to withstand anything, our mental discipline the shield against hardship. Resilience gives us the freedom to shape our destiny.

Developing self-control serves us well throughout life. Those who consciously strengthen their willpower cultivate true inner strength and stay focused on goals even when motivation wanes. They stick to their principles when others don't, and they are less likely to give in to unhealthy urges. Resilient people face challenges head-on instead of relying on quick fixes that simply bury issues for later. They also accept what's out of their hands and instead use their energy to make the most of opportunities and factors still within their control. By choosing to channel their power inward through discipline, they develop the deep resilience that rewards them for the long haul. It's about growing in wisdom and fortitude every day through both ease and struggle.

Problem-Solving Skills

Resilient people turn challenges into stepping stones. They welcome difficulties as chances to learn and develop rather than them as threats.

With a growth mentality, they actively seek constructive feedback and willingly change their approach based on results rather than stubbornly insisting on one path. They face issues head-on by viewing them simply as signs that more information is needed instead of total failures. With open minds, they then think beyond boundaries to find alternative solutions with a resourceful, creative spirit. Growth means change is embraced rather than feared, especially when what's been tried doesn't work out. By harnessing setbacks as problem-solving fuel, you can cultivate optimism and empowerment to achieve your dreams despite life's unavoidable curveballs.

At their core, resilient people approach life from a place of calm determination rather than despair when storms hit. Excuses are avoided, instead focusing on what they can control at the moment. They have an optimism that comes from positive self-talk during hard times, focusing on their strength, not weakness. They welcome challenges as adventures rather than foreign foes, meeting each new experience with mental flexibility and upbeat problem-solving rather than panic. Resilient people tap into their creativity from within, even when under pressure. They see in uncertainty what others miss: opportunity.

It's a mindset we can all learn and apply when tougher seasons come knocking. By aligning our thoughts with reality instead of overreacting, you have the power to transform stresses into steady growth and lift yourself continually to new heights.

Strong Social Connections

While resilience is personal, no one can go through it completely alone. We all need others, even if it's just one or two trusted allies. Our minds and bodies are wired to share good and bad times with people who provide understanding without judgment. Bottling up fears or failures may seem brave, but those emotions often grow toxic over time if left unexpressed. Major life transitions naturally stir up uncertainty that benefits from a wise perspective beyond our own.

Solving problems in isolation isn't how we're wired as social beings. So, even if you're naturally solo-minded, seek out secure communities, mentors, or close friends to listen and offer hope when you're facing challenging seasons. These people will energize you in ways that prepare you to face another day. Your resilience always gets a boost by opening up to caring people, even if just for reassurance now and then that you've got this.

Those who bounce back from difficulties put effort into keeping relationships strong. They nurture bonds with family, friends, and coworkers, so they have caring people around for support when life's uncertainties hit. Rather than wait for problems to damage bonds long-term, they openly discuss tough issues and disagreements before these little issues grow bigger. Resilient people know that keeping communication lines open through good times and bad makes troubles much easier to face in the future. Whether tough situations come down the road or not, prioritizing meaningful connections helps create a support system to lean on through life's ups and downs.

Survivor Mentality and Perseverance

Resilient people have a mindset of empowerment, not powerlessness. They acknowledge difficulty but choose to keep moving forward through tough times instead of feeling paralyzed. Rather than playing the victim role or expecting others to fix their problems, they take ownership of their situation. No matter what challenges come their way, the resilient just keep going, making do with what's available to slowly but surely move in a positive direction each day. Even small steps count! Facing hurdles with determination and positivity makes it possible to continue progressing step by step instead of staying stuck.

This perseverance comes down to conscious decisions, not luck. We build mental toughness by viewing emotions as waves that rise and fall, not as permanent destroyers of hope. When feelings overwhelm you at first, give yourself a break to digest them, and then come back to the situation. Know that beyond short-term upsets lies peace. You've managed stormy periods previously to find clearer skies. Rather than getting pinned down, resilient souls feel what they feel yet still steer toward their goals. Recognizing challenges for what they are—temporary—allows smooth sailing once again after passing through rough patches. You've got this power within you too.

Take a Positive Perspective

Resilient people focus on potential even when others see only doom. They feel real struggles in the present but look for how challenges can make them wiser or bring unexpected good. Even the worst news might lead somewhere hopeful if we look. The strongest among us don't ignore the pain but instead search for how it could better equip them to understand themselves and others going through similar trials. The toughest times often connect people in caring ways, and show our shared humanity if we open our eyes to the rays of light around the darkness. No matter what punches life throws, within every blow lies the power to gain compassion, which lifts both ourselves and those we encounter.

It's normal for sadness, worry, or uncertainty to arise when situations change unexpectedly. However, they make a point to lift themselves out of negative thought patterns that lead nowhere good. The resilient converse kindly with themselves and their loved ones to find a balance between facing hard truths and seeing hope grow even from ashes. While honoring struggles, they look for breakthroughs with determination and care for themselves and others. By being open to both the darkness and the dawn within tough moments, step by step, you can move toward sunlight again.

Growth Mentality

Moreover, the most resilient can roll with life's unpredictable changes. They adapt instead of suffering more from sticking to strict ideas about how things should be. They see obstacles as useful information pointing to new skills needed, not as failures. Perfectionism doesn't hold them back, either. Without ignoring difficulties, they restart with openness and knowledge gained from past mistakes, guided by past experiences showing potential ahead if adjustments get made. Facing challenges means finding ways to gain and improve oneself, not losing hope. Growth happens not despite hard times but often through facing them, adapting approaches, and keeping an open mind.

Emotional Regulation

Understanding and handling emotions well lets resilient people express what they go through in helpful ways, not bottle it up. They see difficulties as natural parts of life, reducing overly strong reactions. While honestly facing peaks and valleys, the strongest also embrace practices like mindfulness, spirituality, and healthy escapes to lower stress when feeling overwhelmed. Through conscious effort over time, resilient people develop their ability to deal with whatever challenges come. Knowing and understanding their emotions serves as useful information for navigating turmoil with care, acceptance, and direction toward growth and connection, even in tough times.

Focusing on the Controllable

The most steadfast tend to stay in their circle of influence, where they can still make a difference, rather than wearing themselves down and thinking endlessly about things beyond their power to change. They don't ignore problems, but they also avoid getting trapped rehashing what they can't directly impact—to preserve their mental strength for focusing on the controllable aspects of their situation.

It takes wisdom to see the line between fixating on worries and constructively facing what realistically can still be steered in a good direction. Resilient individuals direct their efforts carefully toward areas with room for positive change instead of hopelessness. They work on what's within reach today and don't lose time in the present stressing over immutable pasts or distant uncertainties.

Self-Compassion

Those who bounce back treat themselves with kindness instead of harshly judging mistakes beyond their power. They recognize that all people sometimes fall short, and see setbacks as natural, not proof of flaws. Resilient individuals don't condemn themselves for issues outside their control either. They use an understanding inner voice that lifts them when challenges arise, rather than a critical one that intensifies difficulties through shame.

Compassion for one's humanity helps resilient people avoid obstacles that self-blame usually magnifies, leaving us feeling stuck and hopeless. When facing troubles, the resilient offer care and forgiveness to themselves, just as we would comfort a good friend.

Acceptance and Keeping It Real

Those who are resilient face facts realistically but also stand up for change within their control rather than raging against the entire world. They don't dismiss issues with fake optimism or see every difficulty as absolutely hopeless. By adjusting their mindset to the truth, resilient people know everyone has been hurt along the way, yet today's pain doesn't have to limit tomorrow's potential.

They go with life's flow instead of clinging strictly to how things should be and suffering even more from surprises. Challenges provide lessons on extra skills needed for dreams, not proof that efforts are pointless. Facing obstacles provides chances to gain strength, not lose it completely. Resilient individuals grow wiser from hardships rather than stay defeated by them.

Reframing Negative Thoughts

Resilient people are aware of feelings that emerge during hard times, without buying into fear-based narratives of things inevitably falling apart. They nourish optimism to counter worried thinking patterns that lead nowhere. While allowing themselves to feel sadness, hurt, or frustration, they don't accept those thoughts as absolute truth or permanence. They give space and time to process emotions around difficult news without assuming today's troubles define their tomorrow.

They remain open to the possibility of learning, growth, or even unexpected good somehow rising from present hardships. Even when facing difficulties head-on with determination, they maintain gentle open-mindedness to balance perspectives. Resilient people expect to find a way through hardship with strength, perseverance, and heart, believing crises need not crush hope for brighter days ahead. Through challenges weathered with wisdom and care for themselves and others, resilient people go through hardship with a positive yet productive mindset.

Exploring Options

Those with resilience see uncharted territory as a chance to envision new solutions rather than accept limitations. When their usual methods aren't working, they let creativity flow to explore unexplored pathways. They believe unforeseen answers can emerge through open-minded discussion of various options rather than resignation to their fate. With trust in their intrinsic guidance, they confidently refine strategies as situations change instead of becoming rigid.

Living and learning continuously means cultivating flexibility over flimsy plans. Facing shifting circumstances requires fluid adaptation, not inflexibility that breaks under evolving pressures. Growth depends on this ability to modify approaches when one approach doesn't fit with shifting needs. For resilient people, every challenge carries the seed of progress and growth if they focus on options over roadblocks.

Setting Healthy Boundaries

The resilient know how to set smart limits on where they put their time and care. They guard what's within their power while letting go of what isn't. Instead of wearing themselves out and worrying over things they can't change, they guide their focus with sound judgment. Not because other issues aren't important, but to maintain the capacity needed to create real change where they have the direct ability to make a difference.

They recognize humans can't control everything but can optimize what is within their hands to shape. They maximize their positive influence by avoiding exhaustion worrying over things they can't change, even if they are still passionate about larger causes surrounding it. It's about protecting empowerment and impact through selectivity, not dismissal or apathy. Set boundaries, then offer hands extended.

In the end, resilience is an innate, nurtured skill integrating self-reflection, discipline, flexibility, community, empathy, and determination to overcome life's difficulties through any viable avenue. By understanding the perspectives that strengthen us over time, each person gains extraordinary power and inventiveness to turn suffering into purpose. When a crisis strikes, some collapse in blame and hopelessness while others find a breakthrough. This choice is ours. Together, through shared struggles, let our resilience show how even in life's hardest situations, strength, wisdom, and hope can form something beautiful. Hardship need not shape your fate; with care for yourself and others, your destiny remains in your hands to shape as you brave each test and storm. Where there is life, there is possibility. Our journeys continue.

The Resilience Ripple

Cultivating resilience as a daily practice can massively improve your overall emotional health, far beyond just bouncing back from occasional difficulties. When you make it a priority to build this skillset, it provides powerful protection against internal struggles like anxiety or depression during life's roughest patches. The research is clear: developing resilience significantly boosts well-being (Idris et al., 2019). Challenges are inevitable, but they don't have to overwhelm us. By incorporating resilience-building habits into your lifestyle and understanding how they strengthen mental fitness long-term, you gain the capability to roll with life's changes flexibly while guarding your wellness. This allows you to benefit from setbacks instead of crumbling under them. Prioritizing resilience means preparing our spirits to emerge from any storm stronger and more grounded.

When we take time to understand the proven mind and body benefits of resilience, it provides fuel to proactively prioritize building this skill, rather than just developing it unprepared through tough times. Studies clearly show the many ways resilience pays off, like greater happiness, lower stress levels, and quicker healing (Cohn et al., 2009), (Tugade and Fredrickson, 2004). Learning how resilience directly boosts our quality of life, health, and even longevity empowers us to fit more practices into our routines that nourish our resilience. Taking good care of our mental wellness powers us through any storm. So, let's explore some of the amazing ways resilience strengthens our spirits, reduces wear and tear on our system, and even lengthens healthy years ahead. Knowledge is power, and over time this power can change our daily choices for the better in small, potent ways. Our resilience is a life investment worth making.

Enhanced Coping Abilities

At its core, developing resilience strengthens our ability to face painful challenges, changes, and uncertainty in a healthy way. When difficult times like loss, transitions, health issues, or relationship issues might otherwise cause us inner turmoil, resilience skills help lift our mood and resolve from within. The resilient mindset empowers us to summon courage and hope from our inner strengths rather than relying solely on external fixes. This allows us to stay balanced even when disruption throws our usual routines off course. With resilience as our foundation, we can weather life's storms with confidence from the driver's seat of our emotional well-being.

When dealing with new or difficult situations, people struggle if they cannot effectively understand and work with their emotions. However, building resilience helps us adapt flexibly and even find opportunities in challenges. Facing hard times is easier when we can thoughtfully process uncomfortable feelings, changes in plans, and sadness—skills that make us stronger over time. Resilience gives us the ability to take hardship in stride so we can continue moving forward healthily.

Reduced Risk of Mental Health Disorders

Did you know that more than 40 million adults in the U.S. are facing anxiety disorders (Booth, 2023)? That's why it's crucial to build resilience, which protects against issues like anxiety, PTSD, depression, and addictions (Dhungana et al., 2022). These conditions sometimes develop when people try to cope with strong emotions all alone as life gets overwhelming. On the other hand, resilient people know it's healthy to ask for help from others when going through tough times. They understand that feelings of shame about needing support are misplaced. Instead of bottling up stress, a resilient mindset makes it easier to talk through intense emotions constructively. Seeking help keeps difficulties from snowballing out of control, preserving good mental well-being even when facing challenging periods.

When dealing with grief and loss, opening up about our pain and experiences with people we trust can help us heal. Through sharing our stories, we can make sense of difficult times and find new reasons to carry on. But resilience means not just waiting for wounds to heal passively over time. Bouncing back from hardship takes active effort on our part. By taking positive steps like embracing new goals or helping others, we recover by moving forward rather than standing still. Facing struggles with determination and community support allows us to grow stronger rather than letting difficulties overcome us.

Promotes Positive Adaptation

Rather than just getting by when tough times come or hoping the effects will fade over time, truly resilient people can experience positive change during and after hardship by choosing to learn from challenges. If we use setbacks as opportunities to develop greater self-awareness, compassion, and life wisdom, struggles can become a source of personal growth. Resilient individuals often see troubles as a chance to gain fresh insights and priorities that help them find deeper meaning and purpose.

While difficulties are never welcome, cultivating resilience means we can still benefit from periods of adversity. By consciously reflecting on what new understandings or strengths we can draw from even rough soil, we can plant seeds of improvement through experiences that might have once felt barren.

Supports Overall Emotional Wellness

Several behaviors can protect our mental well-being and prevent conditions like depression if practiced regularly. Things like slowly facing what scares us, mending relationships before major damage, adapting to life's natural changes, and asking loved ones for help with major problems—all part of building resilience—can make a real difference. Our emotional wellness develops a lot like our physical health, which requires healthy activities maintained over time.

Just as we watch what we eat and exercise, we must be aware of looking after our inner state by thoughtfully handling whatever difficult situations come our way. While painful or unlucky events are outside of our control, we can influence how disrupted or distressed we become through small, intentional efforts each day. These exercises strengthen our resilient muscles and leave us better equipped to face the next emotional challenge. Taking good care of our mindset provides stability during life's unavoidably bumpy parts.

Facilitates Recovery From Trauma

Many people who have endured unimaginably difficult experiences, such as war, natural disasters, or violent attacks, consistently show that possessing resilient qualities profoundly influences how they cope with trauma. Those who bounce back tend to develop a deeper state of well-being compared to before the event, while others, unfortunately, suffer ongoing issues. Something protective resides in resilient thinking and habits, which enables those who possess it to make it through crises with strengthened purpose and perspective, rather than having problems like PTSD take over. At those crossroads between lingering effects and recovery, resilience appears to hold power over whether a curse becomes a blessing. These remarkable transformations remind us that how we process even life-shattering circumstances makes all the difference.

Improves Quality of Life

Research shows people are happier, feel more fulfilled, and are more thankful for life when they can handle difficult times in healthy ways (Kushwaha et al., 2022). So many struggle unnecessarily because they lack methods for coping with changes, losses, uncertainty, or evolving situations that leave them feeling off-balance. Having resilience is like fuel that keeps us on an even keel, even through rocky passages. Just like looking after our bodies needs good fuel, our emotions do too. By learning new perspectives and responses now, we equip ourselves to maintain well-being when life gets messy like it tends to. With the practice staying strong and adaptable, we keep our emotions and well-being under control even when circumstances aren't.

Resilience Realities and Myths

There are some misunderstandings around building resilience that can hold us back. Let's clear up some myths about resilience and gain a better grasp of what makes us stronger in the toughest of times. Whether we realize it or not, becoming more resilient starts from within through small yet meaningful daily practices, despite life's unpredictable changes. Focusing on what we can control allows us to weather whatever challenges come our way while maintaining an even keel.

Misconception 1: Resilience is built in only one way.

Reality: There are many paths to building resilience. While some find meditation, exercise, or therapy helpful, others build resilience through finding meaning and purpose, developing self-confidence, fostering connections, or learning coping techniques. An individualized, multi-faceted approach works best.

Misconception 2: Resilient people go it alone.

Reality: Connecting with others provides vital social support for resilient people. Whether confiding in trusted friends and family, participating in community groups, volunteering to help others in need, or building other meaningful relationships, connections help buffer stress.

Misconception 3: The focus of resilience is managing negative emotions.

Reality: While processing difficult emotions has its place, positive emotions, and experiences more strongly predict resilience by broadening perspectives and building resources for coping. Focusing on enhancing hope, meaning, gratitude, inspiration, awe, joy, and other positive states builds resilience over time.

Misconception 4: Resilient people power through stress and illness.

Reality: Pushing oneself in the face of physical or emotional exhaustion often backfires, worsening health and diminishing resilience over the long run. Resilient people know the importance of rest and self-care to promote recovery and balance. Taking a break or reducing responsibilities during times of increased stress preserves resilience.

Misconception 5: You either have resilience or you don't.

Reality: We all have innate resilience, which varies with circumstances and can grow substantially. Resilience involves behaviors, thoughts, and attitudes that anyone can learn and develop through daily practice. Intentionally using resilient strategies during everyday challenges builds resilience muscle over time (Davis, 2016).

Misconception 6: People are born resilient.

Reality: While genetics play a partial role, resilience stems largely from experiences and environments. Nurturing relationships, modeling resilience, promoting education, facilitating social connections, and teaching coping skills, especially in early life, provide the foundations for developing resilience despite adversity. No one is simply born resilient without the benefits of caring support systems.

Misconception 7: Resilient people don't let things bother them.

Reality: Even highly resilient people still feel stressed or upset when life gets difficult. Healthy resilience means acknowledging and accepting difficult thoughts and emotions rather than suppressing them. Processing feelings by talking to trusted friends, journaling, or exploring counseling builds coping capacity over time by learning from challenges.

Misconception 8: Resilience is always good.

Reality: While generally positive, extremely high resilience could at times reflect desensitization or an unwillingness to realistically weigh risks and setbacks. Over-resilience can also manifest as a refusal to seek or accept help. Balancing resilience with flexibility and a grounded perspective allows appropriate responsiveness across diverse situations. Absolute resilience may hinder recognizing when an alternate approach works best for positive outcomes.

Misconception 9: Resilience is about bouncing back.

Reality: More than just recovering, resilience involves growing stronger in the face of challenges. Resilient people build self-knowledge regarding what gives them purpose and meaning in life. Recognizing these inner strengths bolsters confidence to proactively navigate difficulties, drawing from experience to transform obstacles into opportunities.

Misconception 10: It's entirely up to you to build your resilience.

Reality: While personal qualities contribute, environmental factors substantially enable resilience capacities. External support systems provide essential nourishment, education, and stability early in life. Ongoing positive community interactions, professional opportunities, health resources, and safe living conditions allow people to enhance their inner resilience. Combined social connections and personal development empower growth.

Misconception 11: Asking for help means you're less resilient.

Reality: Seeking help demonstrates self-awareness, courage, and foresight to avoid getting overwhelmed amid crises. Prioritizing well-being requires acknowledging limitations and utilizing available resources as necessary. Far from being a weakness, appropriately asking for and accepting assistance to address challenges is itself a resilience-building practice.

The great news is that resilience stems largely from acquired skills, not innate qualities. Through developing personalized stress management techniques, fostering supportive relationships, embracing growth mindsets, and practicing positive coping strategies over time, anyone can cultivate greater resilience even amid adversity. Rather than a fixed trait, resilience unfolds daily through enhancing awareness and purposefully taking small steps to broaden your capacities.

Chapter 2:
The Biology of Bouncing Back—How Our Bodies Foster Resilience

Whether recovering from illness or enduring traumatic loss, we all face times of difficulty. Yet some people navigate these obstacles with grace, while others crumble, overwhelmed by the strain. Why do some individuals appear more resilient in the face of crises? What underlying factors allow them to adapt and carry on?

Resilience depends on far more than just attitudes and behaviors. Our very biology influences how we handle and bounce back from adversities. Exploring the science behind resilience provides clues for cultivating this vital capacity within ourselves.

The good news is resilience arises from multiple interacting systems within the body and brain developed over time through evolution. While genetics play a partial role, science confirms that environments and experiences substantially shape resilience, through altering brain connectivity and stress hormone regulation (Parmar, 2022; Ellwood-Lowe et al., 2022; Swaminathan et al., 2023). Unlike fixed personality traits, resilience stems largely from external and modifiable factors.

Having a strong immune system is an important part of resilience. Our bodies need to be able to fight off germs and recover quickly from illnesses or injuries to handle life's stresses. People with weakened immune systems experience more frequent sicknesses, which zap their energy at the same time they're trying to emotionally cope with an illness. Making consistent efforts to take care of ourselves through things like regular exercise, healthy eating, enough sleep, and reducing excess stress all serve to strengthen our immunity over the long run. When our bodies are well, we have more capacity left over to get through rough patches without feeling worn down. Taking good care of our health and immune defenses builds resilience for facing challenges on both the physical and mental levels.

Having a healthy heart and circulatory system also contributes a lot to resilience. Beyond just carrying oxygen and nutrients where they need to go, our cardiovascular system also influences how well-equipped and clear-headed we feel during stressful times. When our heart and blood vessels aren't functioning properly, we tend to feel drained, and our thinking becomes murkier, making it tougher to handle sudden problems. Making consistent choices for cardiovascular fitness through things like walking, running, or other moderate exercise helps ensure we have energy reserves to power through tough emotional periods without losing focus or composure. Taking care of our hearts provides inner toughness to see challenges through without wearing them down.

The way our brains are wired and communicate also plays an important role in resilience. Our neural pathways constantly change based on what we go through, with neuroplasticity allowing the brain to rewire itself actively. More resilient people have brains that flexibly adjust pathways and synapses in response to difficulties while maintaining smooth signaling between brain regions. Specifically, more integrated and balanced communication links survival centers with areas overseeing focus and high-level thinking. Though some resilience may run in our genes, experiencing nurturing surroundings early in life helps sculpt a brain structure that remains adaptable and coordinated. Such a brain structure leaves us better able to bounce back through fostering enriching and supportive bonds. Even as adults, we can help keep our minds resilient by pursuing stimulating activities and relationships.

Getting quality sleep deserves focus, as it's vital for our resilience. When we rest, important recovery activities rebuild our immunity, nervous system, hormone levels, and energy metabolism—all of which help us handle whatever changes life brings. But not sleeping well seriously harms our resilience. It depletes our mental sharpness and physical reserves, leaving us weakened during stressful periods. Prioritizing sleep each night plays a big role in maintaining our natural resilience and strength. It's while we sleep that our body entirely refuels and refreshes its ability to take on challenges with alertness and energy, ready to cope with what's ahead. Neglecting sleep undercuts how well we can bounce back from difficulties.

Of course, biological factors alone cannot explain resilience, nor do they promise protection against all misfortune. However, understanding the physical machinery from which resilience arises provides a starting point for understanding, allowing us to consider ways we might bolster our capacity to recover during hardship.

The Resilience Matrix: The Brain-Body Connection in Resilience

Bouncing back from tough times involves way more than just having a positive attitude. The ability to adapt in the face of stress or crisis relies on a bunch of complicated processes happening in both the mind and body. Even though it might seem like resilience depends mostly on how we think, feel, and act, the physical part plays a huge role too.

Understanding exactly how the brain and body connect to create resilience gives power. Having this information allows for customizing the best personal plan for strengthening the ability to bounce back from hardship. So, while the science behind resilience can get technical, grasping some key points goes a long way toward building this critical skill.

First up, let's define resilience as being flexible and able to regain mental and physical balance during hardship. Resilient people can adapt to evolving circumstances, regrouping their resources to heal and keep thriving. This means managing both the mental stresses and physical strains that tough times churn up.

The brain and body are interconnected through the nervous system and hormones. What happens to one directly impacts the other, whether instantly or over time. Let's break this brain-body resilience matrix down.

Stress starts in the brain, which senses a threat and sends signals via nerves and chemicals. These messages race to other parts of the nervous system, setting off reactions. Heart rate speeds up, breathing gets rapid, muscles tense, and blood pressure fires up. Immune cells activate while digestion and tissue repair slow temporarily until the danger passes.

This revved-up state fuels a quick reaction in an emergency—great for cavepeople escaping predators! But modern threats tend to be stressful situations rather than hungry lions, so all that amped physiology either keeps circulating or leads to exhaustion. Bathroom breaks get skipped, poor food choices happen, and headaches or worse troubles brew.

That's just the physical strain. The ongoing mental anguish and concentration on the stressor spin the brain into an endless loop. People dwell on worst-case scenarios or self-blame instead of taking constructive steps. Without relief, the spiral continues downstream, zapping even more physical and mental energy. It's a nasty cycle!

But resilience breaks the loop! Having appropriate coping skills allows the nervous system to chill out faster after stress activation. Finding meaningful purpose in the situation or drawing on lessons from past success helps reframe the brain's perspective. This gives the pit in the stomach time to unwind and the aching muscles time to relax.

A resilient brain stays rationally responsive when difficulties hit, sending carefully calibrated alerts rather than overblown distress signals to the body. Levelheadedness avoids unnecessary exhaustion and harm over the long term. Quieting worried thoughts prevents churning stress chemistry and continuous strain.

With practice, guiding the brain toward a resilient mindset creates helpful hormones and immune chemicals that then circulate to nourish tissues in need. Troubles still hurt, but the pain passes quickly. Growth opportunities even emerge from the mess!

Beyond biochemicals, purposeful resilient behaviors like moving the body, finding humor, or expressing emotions also soothe stressed physical systems. These healthy outlets break tension while stimulating positive neural connections. And just as the mind can positively impact physiology, the body likewise calms an anxious mind. Techniques like controlled belly breathing or adopting empowering postures reliably ease distress.

This two-way resilience street between brain and body explains why lifestyle habits like nutrition, exercise, and sleep so profoundly influence mental health and healing from hardship. Fortifying that foundational terrain makes handling difficulties much more doable. Alternatively, an already depleted system has few reserves, so even minor disruptions provoke major breakage, like the last straw breaking the camel's back.

The big takeaway here is that physical health and mental and emotional well-being intertwine, relying on each other. Resilience, therefore, requires holistically supporting both realms. Keeping critical body systems strong and flexible makes maintaining a resilient frame of mind easier when push comes to shove. Cultivating positive coping strategies gives the physical side a much-needed respite to re-energize. Play to your strengths for maximal bounce-back capacity!

The Role of Genetics in Resilience

When it comes to handling life's curveballs, genetics do play a part in why some people cope better than others. Specific genes impact how sensitive we are to stress and how well we bounce back from difficult situations. But here's the big news: these genes only set the stage, not the whole story! Day-to-day lifestyle habits and surroundings also shape resilience a ton.

Genes are like instruments, while lifestyle and environment act as the musicians. A good violin supports sweet jams but needs a skilled player to create tunes through dedication to the craft. The same goes for resilience capacities, which come from a mix of inherited traits and life experiences. Let's break it down.

Certain genes control the production of key chemicals that affect how we react to stressors and regulate emotions. For example, serotonin levels in the brain strongly influence mood and nerve cell connections. People inheriting genes that reduce serotonin efficiency tend to be more anxious and handle pressure less smoothly.

However, lifestyle habits like exercise and nutrition boost serotonin for better regulation in response to difficulties. Social support also calms nerves via hormones that counteract genetic sensitivity. Just as muscles strengthen with training, purposefully managing stress reshapes biological resilience over time, including genetic expression.

Another chemical called brain-derived neurotrophic factor (BDNF) encourages new neuron growth while helping existing brain cells survive. Low BDNF is associated with increased depression and anxiety risks, especially during high stress. External enrichment from things like learning, problem-solving, and positive social interaction releases extra BDNF despite genes that normally don't produce as much.

Beyond influencing amounts of specific resilience-related chemicals, some genes impact overall stress sensitivity at a cellular level. Differences in receptors detecting threats and triggering alerts can make some people extra reactive, while gene variants regulating the hypothalamic-pituitary-adrenal (HPA) stress axis alter recovery times. High sensitivity takes more effort to cultivate resilience skills that turn down overactive alarms.

Meanwhile, certain gene types limit hardiness against the wear and tear of chronic strain. Over time, stress piles up damage if adequate recovery fails to happen. Variations also exist for genes, controlling inflammation and immune defenses involved in healing processes. Together, these affect how much backing we need when adversity strikes.

So, what does this all mean for becoming more resilient with the genes you've got? First, understand that your abilities partly depend on the hand genetics dealt you initially. Your temperament, sensitivities, and physiological bounce-back capacities relate to this inherited resilience "guide" so to speak. There is no need to toughen out discomfort levels beyond your wiring.

At the same time, the choices you make daily, whether through thoughts, behaviors, lifestyle, or environmental adjustments, significantly impact how well you cope with hardship versus crack under pressure. Every small step toward managing stress actively shapes gene expression toward resilience capacities. Genetic predisposition alone does not seal your destiny!

For a real-life example, take the inherited risk for mood or anxiety disorders. Early-life nurturing care, healthy community connections, and strong coping skills taught and modeled by resilient caregivers can profoundly buffer genetic vulnerabilities. Regular exercise provides neurochemical mood boosts, while good sleep habits manage sensitivities, both of which are extremely protective.

Even epigenetics—how lifestyle tweaks turn gene volume up or down—plays a role! Constant small positives truly trim cumulative life stress. So, next time you face life's harder moments, remember genes only pen the first resilience draft defined by heredity and early life environment. You hold the red pen, making edits daily through your current lifestyle and surroundings. With consistent touch-ups, anyone can revise their resilience script toward the story they want. Genes might load the gun, but you ultimately pull the trigger!

Neurobiology of Resilience

When facing seriously stressful stuff, how well we endure, adapt, and bounce back depends a lot on what's going on between our ears. The brain controls how we appraise and react to difficult situations, like an air traffic control tower managing threats. Certain parts specialize in recognizing risks, triggering alert signals, regulating emotions, or enabling thoughtful responses. How these centers communicate and coordinate resilience reflexes varies among people.

The core brain areas mobilizing emergency resilience action are the amygdala, hypothalamus, locus coeruleus (LC), and sympathetic nerves. Think of them like an armed forces unit, initiating the brain's rapid deployment sequence when adversity strikes. Even perceiving threat cues like angry voices or reading scary headlines can activate the neural alarm system before we consciously register the reasons why.

When sensing a challenge, the amygdala sparks up, shouting "Red alert, red alert!" to other zones. This almond-sized area of our brain handles primal emotion processing, specializing in fear and anger responses. It compels us to act now with limited information, which is great for escaping immediate dangers but often overreact when threats seem uncertain or complex.

Next, the hypothalamus receives amygdala warnings, firing up sympatho-adrenal forces via the LC. Nicknamed the "urgent action" dispatcher, this node cranks up norepinephrine levels to maximum, surging blood pressure, adrenaline, cortisol, breathing, and heart rates to prepare the body and mind for crisis management. Great for short-term fight-or-flight needs, but too much of it in the long-term strains health.

Simultaneously, the LC broadcasts to widespread brain networks, saying "To battlestations!" and grabbing attention resources. The LC vigilantly scans for relevant threats and risks but often misses nuance. Relying solely on this emergency threat response leaves minimal mental bandwidth for creative solutions. Resilient brains stay aware but evaluate situations more carefully before leaping to worst-case scenarios.

That's where smart resilience leadership regulates impulses, considering options from a broad perspective before reacting. These chiefs include the hippocampus, prefrontal cortex (PFC), and calming neurotransmitters like GABA and serotonin.

The hippocampus specializes in contextual details, contrasting past patterns with present experiences. This knowledge allows us to respond appropriately to specific circumstances, not just generalize danger. Resilient people consult their hippocampus for wise precedents. Trauma or chronic stress can hamper its contributions, undermining its power to accurately judge our situation.

Meanwhile, the PFC oversees executive functioning, serving as a disciplined coordinator, sage advisor, and skilled communicator directing resilience operations. It overrides impulsive habits and evaluates situations comprehensively, all while orchestrating solutions collaboratively with other brain units. When the PFC leads carefully and with wisdom, resilience flows intelligently even during turmoil.

Here's the game-changer, though: the brain continually rewires itself in response to experiences! This neuroplasticity allows resilience skills to keep developing, despite initial biological challenges. Neural pathways adapt through repetition. With consistent lifestyle and mindset practices, we sculpt more balanced, responsive threat detectors and expansive, discerning resilience leadership. In short, how we use our brain shapes its structure and abilities!

For example, by intentionally cultivating optimistic perspectives while managing anxieties with healthy outlets like music, exercise, or talking with friends, serotonin flow increases. This feel-good chemical balances worry centers, strengthening connections between thoughtful inspirers in the PFC and freaked-out reactors like the amygdala. Over time, even genetically anxious people develop more resilient brain wiring.

Similarly, purposefully focusing attention on positive goals and taking constructive actions to overcome difficulties builds nerve cell pathways for flexible, pragmatic coping styles. Self-motivation and healthy distraction techniques reinforce connections between PFC and reward centers. This gives budding resilience and fertile soil to take root. Even natural pessimists can gradually reorient their neural proclivities with a commitment to growth.

In essence, our brains constantly evolve based on experiences. While genetics provide initial resilience capacities, dedicating ourselves to positive practices—especially when stresses hit—grows stronger neural patterns and intelligent responses bit by bit. Where we place our attention directs neuroplastic changes toward skillful resilience leadership or impulsive overreactions. Keep an eye on the prize for progress!

Environmental Influences on Resilience Development

Bouncing back from tough situations depends partly on individual attitudes, behaviors, and biology. But don't underestimate how much the world around us shapes resilience capacities! External factors like family bonds, community cultures, or even neighborhood safety play huge roles in handling life's curveballs.

Understanding how environments and experiences can bolster resilience even with the same genetic risks reveals pathways for purposefully developing stronger backup power as needed. Let's explore by considering Carlos, who transformed early vulnerabilities into later victories by gradually surrounding himself with resilience-building influences.

From birth, Carlos' family struggled severely in a financial sense in their rural community, often unable to afford enough food or stable housing for him and his six siblings. His father frequently erupted with alcohol-fueled rage after work, while his mother battled chronic depression. Isolated and without support systems or schooling, Carlos lacked the tools to process constant violence and neglect at home.

Genetically, Carlos inherited higher sensitivity, feeling threats intensely while recovering slowly from distress compared to his peers. Attempting to avoid further trauma, he grew insular and distrustful. A cycle of unstable living conditions matching his neural sensitivity towards volatility left Carlos with minimal internal or external resilience reserves by adolescence.

However, Carlos' natural intelligence, curiosity, and hidden determination inspired dreams for a different future. At 15, he finally relocated to a shelter, helping disadvantaged kids access education and being cared for by mentors who taught him emotional coping abilities he had lacked in his childhood. Though at first overwhelmed by navigating fresh academic and social demands, Carlos persevered.

Gradually, the new constructive environment enriched Carlos' intellect and self-confidence, despite early deprivation. Patient nurturing from shelter staff stabilized Carlos' neurological stress systems so he could manage anxiety productively when triggered. Meanwhile, fascinating history lessons and community service projects engaged Carlos' motivation even on difficult days.

After earning his GED, Carlos pursued part-time paralegal work, enabling night classes to launch a psychology degree, inspired to help kids who were denied the same resilience-building opportunities he missed. There Carlos met his mentor, Dr. Alice, who recognized his latent talents and grit, which had partially developed from enduring early trauma. Recognizing the strengths of Carlos' unique sensitivity and drive to transform adversity into service for others, Dr. Alice took Carlos under her wing.

With strong professional backing, Carlos rapidly flourished, developing research skills while co-authoring child psychology papers with Dr. Alice and integrating his lived expertise. Embracing his expanded potential beyond family fate or genetic odds, Carlos soon became a licensed social worker and leading therapist, assisting families like his own from under-resourced neighborhoods.

Today, Carlos guest lectures nationally on cultivating emotional resilience skills in challenging community environments. He founded a nonprofit offering mental health education and youth mentoring for low-income housing areas too, ensuring the next generation of kids had the supportive networks he lacked. Carlos' wife and two daughters now thrive thanks to his healing journey.

While Carlos' early chronic stresses conveyed biological vulnerability, later access to schooling, role models, and meaningful work enabled him to rewrite negative genetic and environmental odds. Targeted guidance shaping mental habits and healthy relationships reshaped Carlos' neural functioning toward resilience. He transformed risk factors into wisdom to pay forward.

Carlos' story demonstrates that outside influences can profoundly mold resilience capacities, especially early in development. But later life improvements still make big impacts too, as the brain stays changeable. Purposefully surrounding ourselves with positive physical, mental, and social enrichment grows empowering habits and brain connectivity correlating with resilience. Our experiences can pave the way for our genes, not just the other way around!

Decoding the Neural Mechanisms Behind Stress Adaptation and Resilience

Let's decode how the brain's structural reaction to strain either makes or breaks resilience. Threat response originates from primitive neural wiring evolved to ensure survival by dodging immediate danger. These brain parts specialize in ultra-rapid action before much thinking. But quick reaction reflexes that once saved our ancestors from predators often backfire in modern complex realities, instead sabotaging stability from chronic stress overload.

The good news? We can consciously rewire our neural resilience pathways by changing lifestyle habits and thought patterns bit by bit, even under high stress. Understanding the key mechanisms at work allows for purposeful influence of the outcome of our neural stress reaction—for breakdown or breakthrough.

Remember the amygdala? Your watchdog for potential threats, programmed millions of years ago in ancient mammals. Shaped by evolution to be hypervigilant, this almond-sized area of the brain receives sensory signals and memories, analyzing them for any whiff of risk. It sparks the body's survival fight-flight-or-freeze instincts before you even realize why. Great for detecting immediate dangers in the wild, but overkill in traffic jams or overstimulating environments.

When the amygdala barks "Danger!" it instantly alerts the nearby hypothalamus, your neurological emergency dispatch, coordinating the body's crisis mobilization response. Instantly, your hypothalamus ignites surging neurotransmitters and stress hormones like adrenaline and cortisol through the bloodstream for rapid reactions while also blocking digestion, immune function, reproduction, and growth processes that are non-essential for immediate survival.

Simultaneously, your brain stem fires off urgent messages through the sympathetic nervous system, telling body organs and muscles to accelerate for imminent action. Breathing intensifies, the heart pumps harder, blood pressure heightens, pupils dilate, and senses sharpen. At the same time, non-essential functions like hair growth or libido either slow down or pause completely. You are now ready for instant feats of fight or flight!

This neural threat response cascade evolved so effectively that it became the permanent architecture our modern brains still inherit. Unfortunately, modern stressors like financial woes, workplace politics, or social media angst tend to be prolonged and ambiguous rather than acute life-threatening situations. So, ancient neural wiring still responds by assuming immediate mortal peril!

Over weeks and months of chronic stress activation, the continual flood of cortisol, adrenaline, and inflammation strains organs that have not evolved for prolonged states of being overwhelmed. Eventually, there is a risk of heart disease, diabetes, infertility, and other stress-linked illnesses. Meanwhile, elevated cortisol and adrenaline also steadily impair cognition, erode positive mood and undermine rational choices, which could curb sources of stress themselves (Dziurkowska & Wesolowski, 2021; Talarico et al., 2011; Karunyam et al., 2023).

In essence, the very neural survival processes intended to ensure longevity and reproduction ironically threaten long-term health during chronic stress. However, the great news is that we can override this destructive cycle by harnessing the brain's plasticity—its ability to structurally reshape circuits toward more constructive behaviors. Resilience training achieves this neural circuit-building every day!

For instance, consistent mindfulness meditation demonstrably enlarges prefrontal cortex regions. These regions are responsible for managing executive functions like discernment, planning, and impulse control. Simultaneously, it calms amygdala alarm reactivity, so we perceive events more accurately rather than escalating every irritation. Mental composure helps buffer emotional storms by growing neural pathways for flexible, appropriate reappraisal of difficulties.

Likewise, focusing daily on positive aspirations, expressing gratitude, and remembering past problem-solving successes sustain goal-oriented optimism and motivation chemistry even amid continuous hardship. This process of recalling and processing successful problem-solving is known as *hope therapy*. This builds hardy neural foundations for persevering despite life's challenges and focuses us forward constructively.

Social connection practices like group volunteering also fortify brain areas supporting healthy pleasure and self-confidence. Such practices are vital to counter isolation or self-criticism tendencies under stress. By changing habits and mindsets, we quite literally change the flow and dominance of signals between neural networks, focusing on resilience-building over-reactive breakdown. In this way, our actions reshape not just behaviors but the brain structure itself!

The key insight is this: our brain wiring continuously evolves based on experiences, a process called *neuroplasticity*. While early survival mechanisms assume the worst and overreact to uncertainty, purposefully replacing this impulse with growth-focused patterns lays the neural pavement, promoting flexible adaptation and thriving through whatever life brings. Resilience thereby grows every day where we place our attention. Lead your brain wisely, and it will follow!

46

Part 2:

Rebounding Mentally and Emotionally

Chapter 3:
Rising Above—Turning Life's Challenges into Stepping Stones

Life offers no guarantees. At some point, we all inevitably face disappointments, conflicts, losses, or unexpected hardships. These adversities, ranging from minor hassles to traumatic life changes, challenge our capacity to adapt and thrive. How we navigate turbulent times largely defines the path of our lives: toward increasing strength, wisdom, and meaning, or downward into bitterness, isolation, and despair.

Cultivating resilience means experiencing difficulties as potential catalysts for growth rather than unnecessary suffering. With skillful navigation, the currents of misfortune can direct us toward greater purpose and joy rather than batting us from rocky shore to rocky shore.

First, we must understand two key realities regarding adversity. Difficulties serve an evolutionary role in human development, spurring adaptation and creative problem-solving in ever-changing, complex environments. Attempting to avoid life's challenges and uncertainties altogether means missing the motivation and skills gained through overcoming them. Some degree of manageable distress promotes individual and collective resilience.

Simultaneously, however, modern realities often impose senseless, excessive strains from systems of inequality, unsustainability, and scarcity. These harsh strains begin to condition behaviors through needless fear and stress. The magnitude or duration of hardship today crosses the threshold of usefulness into the boundaries of harm for many. Relieving unnecessary suffering allows space for personal and social growth. Both realities deserve acknowledgment and compassion.

How then can we skillfully transform adversities into assets? The strategies here integrate timeless wisdom with contemporary science to allow for facing struggles with strength, hope, and clarity. Think of these approaches as resilient surfing—using understanding, balance, and courage to catch challenging waves and maneuvering skillfully toward the bright shores ahead.

Making space for difficult feelings prevents being overwhelmed by suppressed storms. Processing negative reactions and replacing self-criticism with self-compassion lays the groundwork for clear decisions during crises.

Reframing situations from new perspectives builds motivation, prompting the implementation of solutions toward meaningful goals. Small constructive steps prevent stagnation despite uncertainty, allowing for adaptability.

Acceptance and letting go of bad practices allow for minimizing draining regrets, worries, or resentments when adversity cannot change. Making peace with realities beyond our control preserves energy for enhancing one's life within current circumstances. Forgiveness heals relationships strained during crises, so social support stays strong.

Suffering deserves acknowledgment, space for processing, and human understanding. Together, these prevent isolation while nurturing post-crisis meaning.

Helping others through mentoring, activism, or charity work allows victims to become victors. By passing on hard-won wisdom, people transform pain into purpose. Even intense personal struggles strengthen social ties and progress.

Put simply, resilient surfers flow with life's currents using skill, grace, and grit. We cannot control external storms or eliminate inner turmoil. However, the mindful practices and supportive connections here turn each crest and crash of misfortune into opportunities for gaining wisdom, meaning, compassion, and courage. From there, we can then guide fellow swimmers toward safe harbors together. Use these strategies and lifesaving buoyancy devices during inevitable floods, and your vessel will emerge safer, stronger, and more seaworthy than before.

Challenges that Test Resilience: Identifying Life's Common Adversities

Let's get real—no one escapes dealing with tough times. Challenges arrive for everyone—yes, even happy people with seemingly polished lives on social media! The difference is how we handle the hard knocks life throws our way. Resilience means navigating pain skillfully to minimize suffering and even grow stronger.

Life serves up certain adversities inevitably. The death of loved ones, relationship conflicts, money problems, work stress, and serious illnesses—these hit most people at some point. Physical or emotional trauma sometimes happens unexpectedly too, shattering perceptions of safety.

Reality is messy! But meeting troubles with courage, grace, and grit allows us to gain wisdom from the roughest rides. Building resilience feels very hard during dark passages, but it pays off in the long run. Let's overview key challenges resilience helps manage, so you know what to expect.

Mental Adversity

Mental adversities like anxiety, depression, and low confidence often bring the toughest resilience tests. When our minds turn against us, attacks feel intense and personal. Dark thoughts can challenge getting through each hour when they are severe. Old traumas boiling up again or genetic brain wiring can contribute to but not define futures.

Emotional Adversity

Regulating overwhelming emotions also demands resilience skills every day. Outbursts of anger, rage, excessive guilt, paralyzing grief—these natural human experiences easily overwhelm our best intentions, damaging relationships and health. Balancing inner turbulence prevents worse-brewing storms in the future. This starts with self-compassion, not judgment.

Physical Adversity

Physical limitations, whether temporary illnesses or permanent disabilities from injury or genetics, also challenge resilience profoundly. Coping with exhaustion, pain, and life disruption pushes fortitude and adaptation capacities. Maintaining dignity and purpose despite physical weakness often requires external support too.

Social Adversity

Hellish social situations likewise ignite deep resilience needs. Toxic friendships, bullies for bosses, hypercritical parents or partners—the list goes on! Boundary setting protects us in these scenarios, but that confrontation still stings. Good thing resilience building prevents absorbing others' poison into self-worth!

Financial Adversity

Finally, financial instability crushes many once secure spirits. Job losses or debt strain security for individuals and whole families, demanding major resilience adjustments to prevent long-term damage. Pride, possessions, and old habits cling to us, but adapting flexibly curbs total collapse. Every small saving or support matters.

Now those are just some big-picture adversity domains. Zooming in further, specific diagnoses like PTSD, disabilities, abuse survivor trauma, chronic illnesses, addiction cycles, discrimination, existential crises, and more, profoundly test human resilience on top of everyday issues.

The sheer weight of challenges could depress anyone if viewed as impossible barriers. But remembering that resilience develops through exposure to manageable doses of hardship reframes each difficulty as an opportunity. Effort and guidance cultivate skills over time, just like strengthening muscles through resistance training. What first strains us later becomes strength!

So, when confronting current or future troubles, fully acknowledge the distress. Suppressing helps no one. Then lessen self-criticism about struggles. Life's raw; we're all works in progress. Next, summon your grit and get crackin' on building whatever skills shore up those cracks the best. Small steps forward every day pave the resilience road. And remember people who have been there before provide the best torch-lighting routes from previous storms. This too shall pass!

Overcoming Life's Common Adversities

When troubles hit, remember that old saying—smooth seas never make skilled sailors! Resilience develops best by working through manageable doses of choppy waters. Each challenge builds personal wisdom and strength to navigate future storms.

Mental Adversity

Let's start with bearing life's roughest waves—mental health challenges like depression, anxiety, PTSD, or low confidence. These tidal waves flood even sturdy minds sometimes. But resilience skills offer solid life rafts before one's whole identity sinks. Reaching out early for support keeps distressed from having a final say.

Counseling, whether talk therapy, small group sharing, or coaching, provides guided recovery through turbulent emotions. Trained pros aid in rebalancing strained neural wiring, while prescribed medication assists in the short term. Building a network of understanding ears to uncork bottled feelings prevents explosions too. Even just journaling, art, and music lessen isolation during downhill slides.

Everyday wellness habits also reinforce mental health significantly, especially cutting out excess stressors and toxic people dragging down recovery. Relaxation practices like breathwork, mindful movement, and meditation reboot frazzled nervous systems, so clearer perspectives emerge. The light begins to break through stormy skies. Small, consistent steps forward pile up over time.

Emotional Adversity

Emotional storms also demand resilience and navigation abilities every day. Outbursts of anger, excessive worrying, paralyzing anxiety, or guilt—these experiences easily overwhelm anyone sometimes. But rather than harsh self-blame for acting out under intense duress, radical self-acceptance offers a secure harbor.

Becoming present through gentle, rhythmic activities like walking, dancing, or playing with pets releases pent-up feelings bit by bit. Creative journaling, music, and art unlock emotional logjams when words fail. Confiding in trusted friends allows you to diffuse toxic self-criticism as well. Building emotional intelligence means first showing yourself some gentleness! This lets natural ebbs and flows bloom into manageable opportunities for growth.

Physical Adversity

Managing physical illness, chronic disabilities, or bodily limitations also stretches resilience abilities profoundly. Coping with exhaustion, relentless discomfort, or lost abilities pushes our fortitude and forces major life adjustments. But resilience skills pave paths for fully adapting constructs.

Of course, following professional medical advice ensures appropriate symptom support. Simultaneously, focusing energy on enhancing remaining joys and priorities prevents fixating on limitations. This might include lobbying for accessibility, joining online communities using apps like MeetMe where you can meet new people to combat isolation, or using aided mobility devices to participate in adapted activities. Healthy self-care habits like eating healthy, sleeping well, and adopting relaxing activities into our schedules also aid resilience by preventing additional burdens from stress, poor sleep, and dietary issues. Sometimes, just taking it hour-by-hour when overwhelmed keeps hope flickering. With compassionate grit, one finds the light.

Social Adversity

Hellish social situations likewise demand heavy resilience skills training too! From toxic bosses or jealous friends to hypercritical parents or partners, misery loves company, dragging everyone down. Resilience here means limiting exposure to harmful influences to preserve well-being without guilt.

If relationships feel reparable, clear communication of needs and boundaries helps. Speaking neutrally about behaviors, not character, when requesting change keeps dialogue solution-focused. Counseling guides reconciliation for willing parties too.

However, cutting ties remains wise if patterns continue despite efforts or abuse or bullying occurs. Eliminating cruelty should not require resilience at all, but resourcefully upholding self-worth nonetheless builds confidence to forge healthier bonds. One compassionately moves on, lighter.

Financial Adversity

Financial instability equally devastates security previously taken for granted. Losing income means reshaping priorities and habits. But resilience views pitfalls as opportunities. Mining hidden talents or passions offers a renewed sense of meaning when old identities crumble.

Of course, budgeting tightly, getting coaching, and applying for assistance cushion crises initially. But a long-term growth mindset also empowers perseverance. Maybe this nudges a career pivot toward a more fulfilling job, less susceptible to the next downturn. Silver linings emerge if one is open to radical self-awareness about what truly matters most, beyond just survival. Our essence persists, whatever external conditions.

The key across all domains remains upholding compassion and hope daily. Look back at how far you have already come, at the resources found to overcome past adversities before this one and know more awaits within. Keep eyes on bright horizons, using each challenge to build skill. Land ho!

Personal Stories of Overcoming Adversity

Nothing proves resilience better than real people walking the walk through raw, messy life changes. Let's get inspired by fellow travelers who turned treacherous terrain into growth journeys using compassion, hope, and grit as compasses.

Maya's Story

First, meet Maya, who is always hustling multiple gigs to support her young son as a single parent. Despite exhausting hours, her optimism and humor lit up every room—until the headaches began. Within weeks came the terminal brain cancer diagnosis, crushing dreams instantly.

Bedridden rapidly by seizures, treatments, and depression, Maya's upbeat spirit dimmed. Her sibling stepped in temporarily to care for Maya's understandably confused son. "My body and mind betrayed me," she explains. "I felt simultaneously isolated yet completely dependent, losing the independence and dignity I valued most."

Inching back from despair's edge started with embracing support from every little offer—friends sitting bedside, volunteers delivering meals, or spiritual leaders visiting to chat. "I learned to receive grace and to forgive my limitations. My community carried me through the darkest times."

Bit by bit, Maya rediscovered sources of meaning and purpose despite her physical decline. She recorded bedtime stories for her son, wrote letters to loved ones for later years, and even sang favorite hymns from childhood with church members over video calls. "Reconnecting to my essence, my core spirit, enabled me to find tiny joys each hour."

Over a year later, Maya continues to defy her original grim projections. No longer able to work formally, she hosts support groups for fellow patients online and offers compassion mentoring for distressed teens. "My adversity opened unexpected doors by forcing me to honor emotional and spiritual needs as much as physical ones. Now I gift that wisdom forward."

Emma's Story

Meanwhile, Emma grappled with profound identity loss after her anxious husband abruptly left their decade-long marriage overnight without explanation—just weeks after Emma sacrificed a promotion to move for his career. "My whole imagined future collapsed," she explains.

Reeling without financial security or emotional foundation, Emma initially battled constant panic attacks. She fixated on perceived personal flaws and strained to process the betrayal by her beloved family. Hitting rock bottom means facing the fragility of dreams placed on others rather than inner strengths.

Through trauma therapy, career coaching, legal counseling, and faithful friends holding space for her during meltdowns, Emma pieced together the next steps day by day. She secured a modest apartment to stabilize her home life while updating her professional credentials, soon excelling at a more fulfilling job.

Long-held hobbies like tennis and travel revived Emma's spark too, as she rediscovered personal passions apart from partnership. "My adversity catapulted growth I avoided for years by over-relying on one person for purpose and safety, numbing my core wisdom and needs in the process. Reclaiming empowerment was utterly transformational."

Of course, deep wounds remain years later. Despite largely thriving, the loss of family always stings. But Emma turns her lingering sadness into support for single women rebuilding their lives through her volunteer group. "We gain collective resilience by bonding through shared adversities instead of isolating ourselves," she says. "Growth erupts from life's ruptures if you allow new light inside the cracks."

Maria's Story

Finally, hear how Maria, a senior, accepted fast-changing limitations with humor and flexibility, exemplifying resilient grace. She largely managed arthritis, stiffness, and hearing aids—until macular degeneration suddenly blurred her vision dramatically. Unable to drive or read books she had loved since childhood, Maria felt a devastating loss of freedom and hobbies. Soon, walking grew challenging, even with canes.

However, Maria quickly embraced lifestyle adaptations, allowing the enjoyment of lifelong passions through altered means. Friends record podcasts of newspaper articles for Maria to access the daily news she always valued. Book clubs shifted online, utilizing text-to-speech apps to aid her before volunteer visitor services brought human connection directly home.

Getting out remained important for her emotional health, so Maria strengthened her upper body via adapted exercise routines. This allowed her to maneuver new, light wheelchairs herself without relying on others. Clubs welcomed Maria to play bingo or bridge as before, simply adapting tablet game interfaces to be accessible despite vision barriers. "I still dance in my seat!" chuckles Maria.

"Perspective is key; doing life differently doesn't make it less rich or fun. I focus on gaining, not losing, abilities. When parts fail, creativity ignites! Old things become new joys." Ever the coach, Maria shares her resilience through leading senior center workshops on forging social bonds, integrating mobility equipment use, and discovering fresh purpose. "Adversity will grow everyone's abilities if allowed," Maria winks.

The voices of these courageous people put a face to these resilience concepts. They model leaning into the community when individual strength wanes; releasing limiting stories and habits while excavating new wells of meaning and purpose beyond old domains; and upholding core dignity as circumstances shift. Their imperfect but stubborn progress through life's unanticipated adversities lights pathways for all to follow when storms hit. Healing from hurts means we can hold the space for others someday. Each story lights the way universally.

Learning from Adversity

When times get trying, the absolute worst thing to do is to buy into the story that life's out to get you! Adversity might knock us down, but why we fall matters most. Are temporary failures evidence you're broken? Or are they traction grips that strengthen the legs on resilience so you run faster afterward? Reframing tough turns as transformational coaches build grit nobody can take from you!

Viewing troubles as teachers rather than torture allows for waking up to what matters and realigning accordingly. Pressures reveal true priorities and hidden character strengths when reflecting on them. Maybe you discover untapped talents or unexpectedly deep wells of courage under duress. Growth sprouts from the mud if you nurture lessons learned in the messy process. This makes you bulletproof for the next round, no matter what comes.

But how do you hear adversity's lessons over the surrounding noise? Tune into the frequency of growth opportunities by applying a listening ear within. Emotional resilience starts with radical self-honesty, sitting with discomfort rather than dodging it. Consider tensions as invitations, not indictments or limitations. What core fears or false beliefs might current challenges aim to evolve? Then boldly write a new story!

For instance, say a major business failure exposes overconfidence in certain skills but strengths in recouping creative capital elsewhere. Well, losing one identity need not collapse everything if you are building a fresh purpose on more solid ground using humbler, updated insight going forward. Failure itself matters way less than the interpretations about self-worth attached to any loss. Adversity reveals either warnings or doorways, depending on how you frame stories. Walk through it with courage!

Here are some tips for catching growth opportunities in tumultuous life passages:

- First up, feeling bummed by reversals is natural! But don't hand over total power by perpetually playing the victim. See beyond suffering to revelations trying to emerge. Maybe this nudge toward better work-life balance or relationship-communication alignment has long been ignored.

- Next, reset inner critics trying to shame or blame when goals derail. Go easier on yourself for any perceived mistakes, remembering that everyone eats humble pie sometimes. Getting defensive just distracts from making actual progress. Challenges build character, no matter how messy they are. You always have enough.

- Ask yourself often: What is this difficulty trying to teach? What emotions, fears, or obstacles surface for my growth? How might this experience make me wiser, stronger, or more compassionate? Consider every tension as strengthening resistance training for your resilience muscles!

- Verbal processing in a safe community also illuminates overlooked nuggets of wisdom. Other perspectives shine light from new angles on familiar situations. Feedback offers course corrections when you feel lost. Nobody figures life out alone, no matter how independent. Trying times remind us we need each other.

- Finally, look back at previous adversities you overcame, even small wins. Recall the resources summoned then that can help cope this time too. Seeing the progress made builds momentum for the present trials. The past still lives inside, ready for the next victory lap!

So, next time stormy seasons roll in, brace yourself to catch the growth gusts adversity brings. Shift your focus from avoiding distress toward learning tools to transcend whatever comes your way. Building resilience looks less like smoothly sailing untested seas and more like welcoming wild waves to sharpen enduring strength from the inside out!

Blowing bubbles teaches life's greatest lessons. All those slippery orbs have the skill of balancing between breaths without letting worries pop into positivity. The same goes for chasing dreams through adversity's wind tunnels, trying to throw us off course. Constructively catching air currents allows riding even turbulence higher using resilience perspective shifts. Let's break down key bounce-back strategies for facing any bubble-bursting challenges with flexible optimism.

First, define a directional goal. Don't just avoid problems, so that these challenges become growing pains, not pointless pains on the journey there! Know what drives you too—the emotional rewards coming from achievement. Maybe freedom, confidence, stability, or legacy impact await beyond present hurdles once overcome. This purpose fuels perseverance when you want to quit. Regularly reconnect to the vision when fog hits; form feedback from that setback, then rechart the route. Eyes are always upstream!

Next, make a framework flowchart, brainstorming everything you ideally need to do to reach the goal. Plot granular action steps, resources required, motivating milestones, and metrics confirming progress. Draft your dream team roster across personal, professional, and community domains, and be able to plot out support elements too. Even 1,000-mile trips start with roadmaps guiding each turn ahead. Planning prevents feeling overwhelmed when the route gets bumpy.

With ideal scenarios mapped, honestly identify every possible barrier that could realistically arise to disrupt journeys based on past experiences. Name every weakness causing self-sabotage, such as a money shortage slowing momentum, or envious frenemies thwarting cooperation. Strong vision meets a realistic outlook. Pitfalls show where building endurance takes work, so get strategic!

For instance, imposter syndrome draining confidence requires handy self-affirmations countering memories of fear replaying old failures. Perfectionism bottlenecks output and requires partitioning projects into bite-sized increments with mini-deadlines in order to tackle it, building small successes toward final victory. Getting ultra-creative brainstorming solutions this way empowers breakthroughs!

Assuming challenges inevitably come, whatever tactics are tried will keep perspective resilient. Neither sugarcoating struggles diminishing needed growth effort nor catastrophizing hassles exaggerating true threats help. Flow like water around obstacles without judgment when they inevitably arrive. Rigidity snaps, flexibility bends.

Bring an abundance mindset, envisioning resources multiplying into needs like water that overflowing hands cannot hold. Scarcity shrinks experience while generous attitudes find channels where lack seems guaranteed. Choosing grateful optimism sets conditions for synchronous support to emerge if a patiently persisting vision is aligned to purpose.

Wins often come through unforeseen blessings when locked tunnels suddenly crack open.

Rather than resenting adversity, embrace tension as traction, gaining strength and skills you cannot develop unopposed. Resistance today reinforces next-level capacities once obstacles are overcome. Difficulty indicates simply having to adjust techniques, expectations, or the environment—not accepting defeat as the final verdict. After all, every great athlete still fails more than they succeed in practice! See setbacks as feedback clarifying training needed for peak performance when stakes get high.

Finally, reframing situations more positively prevent spiraling downwards from fixed mindsets, judging struggles as evidence of permanent failure or flaws. Setbacks happen inevitably to everyone, even high achievers. But those who persist reshape brain connections neurologically over time, automatically contextualizing challenges as temporary teaching moments rather than self-defining tragedies. This mental flexibility and grit compound breakthrough potential in the long run. Your bubble can reach the skies!

Chapter 4:
The Art of the Comeback—Overcoming Setbacks and Embracing Failure

Setbacks and failures will eventually enter our lives; no one escapes them forever. Heartbreak follows fairytales. Businesses fail despite the hard work and hustle. Physiques are slow despite disciplined training. Financial cushions disappear overnight. Medical mysteries resist diagnoses and cure-alls. Regardless of intent, preparation, or skill, things simply don't always happen according to plan.

We then face an important choice: crumble into depression or rise stronger with hope. Beyond circumstances themselves, our responses determine if stumbles become devastating dead ends or productive springboards launching new paths. With resilience, we can reframe failures as teachers, developing the character, wisdom, and grit necessary to attempt great things. Each redo and restart builds emotional calluses and problem-solving skills to shine brighter as leaders. There are no successful heroes without tough comebacks that transform wounds into wisdom first.

Opposite to popular belief, failure describes an outcome, not an identity. Just because a project or dream dies does not mean you, as a whole person, are forever seen as damaged goods. Loss often says more about timing, resources, and external luck than individual worth. Separating self-worth from specific achievements allows for confidently attempting great things without paralyzing pressure to protect reputations. You can fail many times, but you fail permanently only when you quit trying new approaches informed by your former struggles. Failure, well adapted to, leads to eventual success.

Progress builds up slowly, and persistence pays off more and more over time. Character is built through difficulties that grow greater empathy, wisdom, and faith for the journeys of others. Skills grow through overcoming ever-changing challenges. Persistence builds up like diamonds from the immense pressure that would otherwise crush weaker spirits. While others may immediately view setbacks simplistically as failures alone, resilient souls with clear vision understand failure as an opportunity to grow further.

As long as the heartbeat continues tomorrow into being, possibilities continue to appear. The art of resilient comebacks involves reframing plot twists as allies, not enemies that sabotage happy endings. Lean into the learning failure offers, and grit awaits right around the corner like a phoenix rising from the ashes. Your boldest dreams still live within. But first, you must bravely sustain faith that, though tears linger one night, joy still dawns with the morning light, ever faithful.

Confronting Setbacks and Failures

Let's get real—nobody's winning 100% across the scorecard of life. Sooner or later, plans unravel, dreams fizzle out, and relationships break apart. Failures frustrate us, leaving us questioning whether our efforts add up to anything worthwhile at all. But winding roads still reach destinations with patience. Growth flows through mourning unrealized expectations before awakening to new possibilities. What matters isn't perfection, but perseverance.

Failures commonly leave people feeling crushed and defeated, but challenges and setbacks themselves are completely normal parts of life. The myth of continuous victory sets false standards, creating insecurity. Comparing and highlighting others' wins while hiding personal losses produces envy and self-doubt. "Why can't I just succeed like everyone else seems to?" In truth, everyone faces downfalls; they just share their celebrations the loudest.

Media feeds and milestone announcements rarely showcase behind-the-scenes tears, late nights, and costly mistakes behind fame. Even high achievers rarely win Olympic golds, Pulitzer prizes, or Grammys on their first try. Success is built brick by brick, learning from slip-ups and redirecting efforts. Progress through following passion includes unavoidable failures bravely confronted. Let's drop shallow pressures to achieve unrealistically without struggles; relief awaits embracing imperfection as perfectly normal.

It is defeating when passionate plans fail and dreams die, making us confront harsh reality. Grief and sadness eat up mental energy initially. Frustrations boil down to trying the same exhausted tactics, hoping for different outcomes foolishly. Disappointment stings where pride once believed there was guaranteed success ahead.

As the dust settles, options narrow, sometimes causing overwhelmingly hopeless thoughts like, "I'll just always fail no matter what I try!" Space opens up, asking, "Why even try when my efforts always seem to backfire?" Anger often arises from being dealt a bad hand yet again by fate, despite the best-laid plans. Fear grows, imagining repeated defeat and becoming the norm for endless futures hardened by former stumbles, never quite stuck.

Vulnerabilities surface too, where embarrassment shames us for broadcasting bold dreams that dried up pathetically. Imposter syndrome whispers, "If I were truly competent, none of this would have happened!" Reputations linking entire identities to specific goals crumble when benchmarks slide backward.

Such overpowering emotions understandably lower ambitions that once dared greatly without hesitation. However, redirecting mental energy toward growth and solutions allows for bouncing forward in time. Gaining wisdom from former mistakes often creates future success stories, transforming perspective into prophecy.

First, accept hard times as natural seasons rather than permanent futures defining your self-worth or creating limitations. Take space first to grieve without rushing timelines toward healing. Release tears and recover energy stores through nourishing self-care. Allowing emotional processing prevents burying away the pain, which will only resurface later in destructive ways. Talk through confusion and anxiety with safe supports who speak with empathy, not attacks, in times of vulnerability. Their grounded confidence restores steadier footing bit by bit.

Next, shift focus toward the upside of the situation, the newfound freedom gained through stripping away what didn't serve you well. Failure redirects us from focusing on what isn't working to allowing exploration into new ways and paths. Reflect on core priorities that spark passion and purpose. Then realign efforts to fulfill that deeper meaning independently, regardless of outside validation. Rediscover work, relationships, and habits that fuel a growth mindset through small daily progress. Consistency produces more success than focus on the finish line.

Finally, have faith that setbacks today often prepare you for increased responsibility and influence tomorrow. Handling a little bit of struggle over time earns the opportunity to handle greater things with maturity and wisdom cultivated through earlier struggles. Bouncing back from pitfalls builds emotional resilience, building the courage to attempt challenges out of reach for those fearing any uncertainty or rejection. Consider each loss a temporary lesson toward wild dreams not extinguished deep down.

Failures feel far from fantastic at the moment. But for reflective souls courageously feeling pain and then seeking significance through it, powerful purpose often awakens. In time, a thriving community finds one another, sharing comeback stories and strategies unique to the challenges faced. What the enemy intends to destroy only comes back stronger through redemption. You were made to weather storms without losing your way. Take heart—your most inspiring chapter is still unwritten.

Turning Setbacks into Opportunities

Bouncing back from failures often requires mental strength as much as practical fixes to address what initially broke. Reframing thoughts empowers comebacks instead of paralyzing sadness. Having the courage to start over comes from believing that better futures await beyond painful pasts. An optimistic lens spots opportunities even amid obstacles once deemed completely crushing.

Turning setbacks into springboards first involves identifying the negative mental narrative holding progress hostage. Does embarrassment from public failure build fear in attempting anything bold to avoid repeated rejection? Does self-criticism, minimizing any wins, create imposter syndrome? Do others' careless words claiming, "You don't have what it takes," echo louder than truth rooted in a persistent work ethic, producing results despite challenges faced?

Catching hopeless self-talk and confronting it is essential. Ask, "Is this absolutely true or somewhat overly dramatic given actual circumstances?" Consider more constructive perspectives grounded in reality. "I haven't arrived fully yet but am actively developing skills and strengths daily." Release needless perfectionism about immediate mastery. "My worth remains regardless of any single outcome, high or low; consistent, diligent efforts build up over lifelong timelines."

Replace demands insisting "I should have known better and avoided mistakes completely" with gentler guidance: "I used the information available at the time and am now prepared for future decisions." Failing guarantees nothing except the opportunity to learn. Setbacks prepare capacity for comebacks.

Language frames experience positively or negatively. Notice the words that only keep useless guilt about the past present in our minds. "If only I had worked harder or planned better, this disappointment would've never happened." Ban all-or-nothing words like "always, never, every time" that turn singular situations into entire identities. Thinking that one disappointment means you'll never live up to your potential or can't be trusted with responsibility only makes you disregard the evidence saying otherwise, built up over the years.

Use more accurate, grounded descriptions, allowing balanced self-assessment. "I didn't achieve specific metric targets this quarter but have successfully delivered projects, saving time and revenue through creative solutions regularly." Framing failures as flukes rather than symbols of self-worth empowers moving forward constructively. Progress often requires trial-and-error learning, not linear victory. Destiny unfolds beyond made-up timelines.

Gratitude journaling builds resilience by consistently recording blessings and wins amid seasons of feeling like nothing is going right. List little daily gifts like cheerful greetings from neighbors, accomplished workout sets, completed errands crossed off checklists, and kids mastering math problems once confusing. Nothing is too small or obvious. Counting up steady examples of providing, relationships, and growth clarifies vision beyond temporary setbacks and tunnel vision. Creating a habit of honoring progress attracts increased victories built up over time.

Surrounding yourself with positive perspectives uplifts your morale, which is crucial during times when we second guess our worth. Certain people consistently see in themselves a powerful identity and a rich purpose, regardless of external measures. They speak of hope grounded in spiritual wisdom and empathy. They voice the truth with love, not condescending judgment. They listen compassionately, then gently remind us that better days dawn amid darkness. They fan the embers of passion and skill, making sure that they do not burn out in future tasks. They expect comebacks by redeeming failures as teachers and turnarounds as testimonies to their ability.

Speaking out affirmations combats internal criticism that is only strengthened through tough losses or public mistakes. Phrases like "I am persistent amid this challenge." "I am growing in wisdom and resilience, which will serve me long-term." "I am proud of the character I have revealed through the difficulties I have faced." "My best self is still growing." Repeat touchstone mantras, replacing the ever-present barrage of self-doubt. Scripture verses paint hopeful landscapes, envisioning destiny unfolding in due time. Quotes from history's great overcomers of hardship help us follow in the footsteps of giants. Speaking words the mind can't yet comprehend builds faith and eventually leads to believing boldly.

The power of positivity sustains focus on the good surroundings even when troubles threaten complete distraction. Zooming perspective back from the microscopic fixation on disappointing failure shows us the blessings around us and helps to realign priorities wisely. Suddenly you notice kind gestures, natural wonders, and special connections that far outnumber losses at any given moment. Health, family, and purpose are far more important than any temporary setbacks, seem much less terrible in the context of global suffering. Deep breaths reconnect beauty, still keeping us in the now despite adversity blinding us to it temporarily. The light still shines even when pain stings and the eyes are tightly shut, resisting peace. Healing happens gradually as we open our minds to blessings present all around us.

Bounce Back Better: Techniques and Mindsets for Rising Above Failure

Falling down hurts—no way around it! Scrapes and bruises sting temporarily, showing little mercy. But most small stumbles heal quickly, especially when cared for gently without judgment. The same proves true after failures rock dreams we worked passionately toward accomplishing. Constructive self-talk, lessons learned, and hope ahead heal egos far faster than self-criticism possibly could.

Start by acknowledging feelings honestly; anger, sadness, fear, and frustration always surface when plans unexpectedly unravel. Vent, if needed, to safe supports who allow tears without dismissing emotions as overreactions. Name specific disappointments aloud to release bottled-up emotions. Accepting loss leads to eventual growth while denying truths pauses forward progress.

Floating in failure's wake, practice self-compassion using language you would extend to consoling a best friend in a similar situation. Tell yourself, "We all mess up sometimes. My worth isn't defined by the stumbles along the way." Thank yourself for finding opportunities to adjust efforts enriched through self-discovery. Send kindness to the hurting inner child who still needs encouragement, even when the strong mask we put on as adults pretends to be indestructible. Growth depends on breathing space to process difficult emotions rather than numbing ourselves to them. You were made for more than surviving—for living fully.

Adopting a growth mindset means believing abilities grow through determined diligence over the years, building up into talents honed gradually and eventually mastered. Genius awakens not from some static quality alone but through many small wins toward increasingly bold vision. What once seemed utterly impossible becomes suddenly possible through step-by-step progress built persistently when passion fuels the climb. Where others see failure as the finale, resilient souls see success as still possibly within reach if they adjust course accordingly.

Common thinking traps reinforce limiting perspectives that need to be challenged to develop accurately. Black-and-white extremes like total winning or total failure blind us to the gray aspects of our path toward success. Down seasons make our lives fuller, ensuring a more successful victory. Identity need not be chained firmly to each victory or defeat. Wise insight acknowledges what we perceive as failure as instead selective filters on reality, and important steps toward progress once momentum is regained.

Reframing failure as redirection renews motivation for the next ventures, now made wiser through former struggles. Take rich insights from loss: "What risks revealed the blind spots I need to strengthen?" "Who might I work with that possesses the missing skills I need?" "What passions are reignited now that my former responsibilities were lifted?" "How did the journey itself change my character regardless of whether the destination was reached?" Celebrate the growth you've achieved through failures and the feedback you've learned from them. New paths await, requiring us to find them through introspection.

With balanced reflection, revisit original goals, assessing what foundations proved faulty in framework or timing, before getting rid of it altogether. Revise dreams, counting the continued costs of chasing them without changing reasonable expectations. Some dreams require endurance and decades of development. Others change into alternative pathways connected more deeply to the core essence of what we want, rather than looking for surface-level titles alone. Patience reigns, realizing that seasons change and call for us to adapt, but never to surrender our hope.

Getting connected recovers emotional wells by tapping into each other's mutual understanding. Those dealing with familiar storms shine a light when shadows cover us. Friendships forged in fire know all too well the weight of waiting, yet they also know the beauty rising slowly over time. Shared stories swap truths. Messages such as "Me too!" build belonging and resilience. Who understands better than fellow travelers walking through steep, narrow paths often avoided? Camaraderie multiplies joy and divides sorrow.

Beyond circumstantial significance, bigger meanings make suffering feel less senseless. What perspectives grew, confronting weakness that pride otherwise might have resisted? How will lessons learned help others facing similar crossroads ahead? What new strengths or passions came into view during hardship? Even the worst chapters hold something sacred when we look back on them with grace and courage.

While riding rollercoasters of setback lows and comeback highs, practical self-care bolsters resilience over the long haul. Gentle nutrition and hydration support the health of the physical, emotional, and mental spheres. Rest recharges perspective, often blurred by fatigue and worries. Moving the body boosts energy and brings out creative connections from where they hide. Laughing lifts the spirit. Small habits build stability when everything feels shaky.

Healthy minds avoid personalized failure and self-attacks. Challenges faced say nothing about our inherent worth or identity. Losing one game, job offer, or relationship guarantees nothing about prospects for joy down the line. Ups and downs show our humanity, not the total of all we are or will become in time. Release the weight of the world off your shoulders; growth flows freely only when unburdened.

Mindfulness allows feeling failure's full pain without drowning in it. Name the loss, then intentionally shift attention toward the now. What senses still work—touch, sound, sight, scent? Count your blessings, beloved souls yet present, and opportunities awaiting in the next round. Breathe fully in this given moment. Grieve hard when waves crash, but in between, immerse yourself gratefully in today's goodness.

Building resilience requires reworking thoughts about falling short constructively. Failure indicates actions, efforts, or plans that did not succeed—never self-worth. Mistakes create wisdom, which is applied differently moving forward. Risk and setbacks teach us bigger capabilities to shoulder responsibility and pursue greatness through growth. Imperfect progress still builds up better than no action at all. What transforms life's lemons into lemonade is a proactive, positive perspective paired with determined action toward dreams. Then momentum regains traction step by step—believe it!

Chapter 5:
The Power of the Mind—Cultivating Mental Fortitude for Resilience

Legend tells of two travelers crossing a barren desert on foot, headed to a distant oasis paradise. As the unrelenting sun beat down on them, and without shade or water sources for miles, one traveler hung their head, taking each tiring step while complaining about thirst, fatigue, and sweat. "This journey seems endless!" they muttered angrily.

The other traveler craned their neck, admiring passing wildlife, unique rock formations, and the awe of an endless blue sky meeting shining sand as far as the eye travels. Even as the bag on their back felt heavier by the hour, a subtle yet persistent smile spread across their sun-kissed face. "I wonder what beautiful scenes lay ahead," they thought aloud with sustained optimism.

The first traveler trudged, soaked in gloom, while the second skipped, happily marveling at nature's majesty. Both travel the same uncompromising terrain, facing identical external conditions. However, the inner lens coloring how each traveler perceives and thus experiences the same pilgrimage differs dramatically, all based on their own private outlook.

The tale illustrates that while we cannot always control outer circumstances, the resilient mind keeps power by framing each event neutrally, optimistically, or otherwise. Mental perspective functions as a compass and fuel at the same time, helping us navigate a variety of obstacles and supplying us with sustained energy to continue our trip. With intentional conditioning, our mental muscles strengthen to support flexibility in perception and build deep wells of hope.

How does one cultivate such durable psychological flexibility and optimism? The mind itself proves to be the most powerful tool we possess for developing mental and emotional health and resilience. Hence the proverb, "As one thinks, so one becomes." When harnessed effectively, the mind empowers us to view disruptions through a lens of opportunity rather than defeat.

Those endorsing the fixed mindset view intellectual shortcomings as evidence they fundamentally lacked the necessary smarts to excel in a subject. Thus, difficulty disheartened them, challenges felt threatening, and they avoided risk or effort to shield their self-esteem. Conversely, people embracing the growth mindset interpreted early struggles as indications that an area simply required further skill development through diligent learning strategies. Difficulty signaled a possibility. Setbacks brought determination, not despair.

As you might expect, the growth mindset fostered perseverance and greater overall achievement. Why? The lens through which we perceive adversity shapes our responses in that crucial moment, where we either constructively confront barriers or abandon hope. Our mindset habits begin to develop early in childhood based on influences like caregiver praise styles (valuing effort vs. intelligence). The good news is that neural pathways remain malleable into adulthood, awaiting our intentional reconditioning.

While we cannot control outer conditions or eliminate adversity, we bear full responsibility for mindfully directing our inner lens, which then shapes individual reality. Our mental perspective uniquely colors how we receive each person and circumstance encountered on the path ahead. By intentionally cultivating mental strength, we prepare ourselves to receive all manner of challenges with grace and grit.

Mental Might and Resilience

The most formidable power we possess remains protected behind walls of bone, yet it influences everything we perceive, feel, and manifest. I am speaking, of course, about our complex brain—the command headquarters directing moods, behaviors, decisions, and more based on trained neural pathways. By consciously strengthening our mental muscles, we gain emotional regulation skills, developing personal resilience through storms within and without.

Defining Mental Strength

Mental strength involves a combination of cognitive, emotional, and behavioral habits that support tenacity despite adversity. Those exhibiting durable psychological fitness demonstrate:

- **Emotional regulation**: They navigate unpleasant feelings skillfully without suppressing, overidentifying, or externalizing inner struggles in unhealthy ways during upsets. Mental strength helps restore balance.

- **Confidence in abilities**: The self-assured leverage personal talents and past wins during the pursuit of their goal, rather than folding when challenges arise. They acknowledge areas for growth.

- **Strategic persistence**: Resilient thinking patterns frame setbacks as feedback opportunities. Such individuals remain solution-focused, avoid dwelling on issues, and monitor their frustration constructively.

- **Interpersonal compassion**: Managing relationships respectfully even when disagreeing requires maintaining empathy, communicating needs clearly, and resolving conflict strategically. We need to work together rather than looking at the other person as the enemy.

Psychological strength cultivates the persistence we often associate with resilience by adaptively guiding thoughts, feelings, and behaviors.

Mental Strength and Resilience

Think of resilience as the destination we hope to reach at the end of hardship, and mental fitness as the vehicle carrying us there. Resilience means enduring adversity, then bouncing back unbroken—holding onto composure and hope despite the disruptive changes, blocks, or disasters. Our brain's fitness supplies the fuel that makes forward progress possible when tough emotional challenges threaten to drag us into despair.

Thus, developing mental strength establishes a mindset and supportive skillset, preventing common psychological traps like turning smaller problems into bigger ones in our minds, overgeneralizing setbacks, or obsessing about problems. Such habitual patterns often intensify emotional distress and prevent us from reaching solutions. With psychological strength, we catch ourselves when blowing up small upsets or imagining unlikely worst-case scenarios, so as not to spiral into anxiety. We celebrate minor milestones that might otherwise go unacknowledged if we dismiss anything short of flawless progress.

Think of mental might as the oxygen mask deployed when normal conditions nose-dive unexpectedly. Our minds can withstand far greater discomfort when equipped with practices for checking exaggerated thoughts, preventing emotional hijacking, and adapting behaviors to align values with proper priorities. External chaos may be non-negotiable, but our mental response remains adaptable.

Benefits of Mental Strength for Well-being

Now that we have defined the interconnected interwoven nature between mental muscle and resilience, what are the positive byproducts of developing psychological hardiness?

- **Better emotional health**: Building mental strength directly provides skills for managing unwelcome feelings triggered by adversity in a balanced, constructive manner. This fosters self-confidence in our capability to eventually restore balance after inevitable ups and downs. We gain greater agency by influencing our inner universe.

- **Improved decision-making**: With turbulent emotions somewhat soothed, this creates the mental space needed for gathering key information, assessing options accurately, considering the details, and determining optimal next steps toward resolution. Our choices prove wiser.

- **Greater success**: By avoiding cognitive traps like self-limiting beliefs or perfectionism, we credit ourselves for undertaking smart risks and celebrate small wins that enhance motivation. We should course-correct rather than abandon hope. Over time, these habits build on each other.

- **Healthier relationships**: Managing interpersonal friction requires maintaining empathy, communicating needs clearly, and resolving conflict strategically rather than selfishly avoiding resolution. Mental and emotional regulation prevents burning bridges.

- **Increased self-esteem**: As we accomplish goals once seemingly impossible, become more attuned to personal needs, and cultivate supportive connections, our self-worth reflects these advancements through an expanding sense of esteem, worthiness, and confidence.

- **Enhanced resilience**: With improved positivity, more efficient, and skills for navigating difficulties, we reinforce resilience reserves to utilize when the next struggle strikes—creating a positive loop and building further mental muscle.

- **Reduced mental health issues**: Common conditions like anxiety, depression, or addiction often relate to unhealthy thought patterns, emotional suppression, and chronic stress. Developing robust psychological fitness protects well-being.

- **Better physical health**: Mental and emotional equilibrium yields downstream benefits like decreased cortisol and inflammation, restful sleep, and motivation for healthy lifestyle habits that serve bodily health over the long term.

- **Overall life satisfaction**: With psychological strength developing career advancement, financial stability, meaningful relationships, and purpose alignment—key pillars supporting well-being—we experience greater gratitude, optimism, and peace regarding the life journey itself.

The mind is sufficiently convinced it can achieve whatever picture it holds, so we must be intentional about the visions we rehearse.

Strategies for Cultivating Mental Strength

When hit by strong gusts of misfortune, our psychological framework is supported by mental toughness, which acts as a crucial cornerstone. Just as physical ability develops through the progressive lifting of weights over time, we must exercise mental and emotional muscle groups regularly to foster durable neural pathways that buffer inevitable storms. Now let's examine some important training methods.

Adopt a Growth-Oriented Mindset

Unconsciously, our beliefs shape the way we behave. Those viewing intelligence and talent as fixed and unchanging factors feel threatened by struggle, avoid risk and fold quicker when challenged. Conversely, a growth mindset views abilities as open to growth so long as we pursue knowledge and practice skills. Mistakes become feedback for improvement rather than indications of inadequacy.

Develop Emotional Intelligence

Emotional intelligence (EQ) means accurately identifying feelings arising within yourself and others, understanding their origins, and responding adaptively. Unmanaged emotions often hijack mental clarity when we need it most to resolve issues wisely. Chapter 10 outlines constructive strategies for honing our EQ through self-awareness, motivation, self-regulation, empathy, and social skills.

Set Realistic Goals

Set goals that are challenging but can be done. Accomplishing them, no matter how small builds up your motivation to aim even higher next time. Breaking big projects into smaller steps makes them less scary to try. For each step, be clear about what exactly you'll do, how long it will take, and what help or supplies you need. Tracking your progress along the way keeps you energized. Once you finish a phase, take time to feel good about what you achieved before moving on to the next part. Recognizing your wins, big or small, will help carry you forward.

Practice Resilience

Journal about or discuss with a trusted friend three personal stories demonstrating your resilience during and after substantial hardship. What internal resources, mindsets, and external supports empowered eventual thriving? Regularly acknowledging these strengths combats the brain's tendency to fixate on flaws. We become what we repeatedly think and speak about.

Strengthen Support Systems

Carefully examine whether relationships energize or deplete precious mental resources. Reduce time with those dragging you down; increase engagement with allies championing your growth. We were made for community, so nurture it wisely. Life's journey requires traveling companions who appreciate our full humanity.

Embrace Change as an Opportunity

View change through a lens of interest rather than as a threat. Changes large and small remain a normal part of life. Focusing our perspective on such shifts proves optional, however. Maintain balance mentally by staying present rather than clinging to uncontrollable past memories or unpredictable futures. Flow with life's seasons.

Develop Emotional Regulation Skills

When intense feelings arise, like anger, anxiety, or hurt, pause. Witness the emotion's arrival without judgment, identify any unhelpful thoughts fueling it, intentionally calm your nervous system through soft belly breaths, and then reflect on skillful responses before reacting. It's incredible how much space even 60 seconds of self-awareness creates for preventing reckless words we later regret.

Practice Self-Compassion and Self-Care

Notice critical inner voices and instead offer encouragement, imagining what a beloved mentor would advise in times of failure. Talk to yourself as you might a dear friend in that situation. Set boundaries around restorative sleep, nutrition, and movement that serve your mind-body vessel. You cannot pour from an empty cup.

Step Outside Comfort Zones

On occasion, choose to attempt an activity that creates some nervousness about uncertain outcomes. Start small by driving a new route or eating food you've never tasted. Such manageable exposures to unfamiliar territory wire the brain to associate change with neural reward chemicals. Each adventurous step fosters courage for bigger leaps.

Develop a Daily Routine

Anchor your day with predictable rituals that are always completed, regardless of the chaos going on in your life. For example, upon waking, meditate in silence to ground nerves, move your body energetically, fuel well through whole food, hydrate properly, and review priority tasks you can directly influence. Structure built through reliable habits creates mental order.

Keep Connections Strong

During stressful periods when you may isolate yourself, lean intentionally into community norms like small group discussions, creating art together, exercising side-by-side, or sharing meals with loved ones. Laugh, cry, and brainstorm solutions. Humans function best when they work together. If tense politics arise, redirect gently back to common ground.

Cultivating durable psychological fitness and resilience requires committing to daily practices that strengthen mental muscles, just as athletes condition the physical. What growth step excites you today?

Your powerful mind awaits earnest direction and small, consistent investments toward incredible gains.

Mind Over Matter

Legend tells of two young songbirds, brothers born as orphans and then adopted into different nests. One elder mama bird constantly critiqued their little one:

"Your voice sounds off-key when you sing. Your wings look awkward in mid-flight. Why waste energy trying complex songs?"

The other mama bird cheerfully encouraged their little one:

"You're strengthening your wings more each day! Keep practicing those tricky new melodies. Your determination will help that solo shine in time!"

You can imagine over the years orphan bird gained vocal skills and confidence, soaring to great heights. The power of our perceived mental narrative proves self-fulfilling. Resilience requires a growth lens to see possibility, whereas a stiff mind frames limitations. Let's see how to cultivate this important mindset.

The Power of a Growth Mindset

Individuals demonstrating a growth mindset operate from an empowering narrative that their skills and even intelligence itself can always expand through determined, strategic effort. Brains continue to be open to growth across our lifespan. Neurons forge new connections, enabling capability growth when we expose ourselves to novel ideas while also committing to deliberate and consistent practice.

Perhaps you accept intellectually that dedication enhances achievement, as evidenced by masters of their fields like athletes, musicians, scientists, and so on. However, when facing personal shortcomings, a common reflexive inner voice whispers criticism attacking self-worth rather than affirming the learning process itself. Paying attention to this negative self-talk and reframing it through a positive lens is important. Instead of focusing on the fact that you aren't at your goal yet, look at all the progress you've made toward it, and know that you will make it eventually.

There are two primary reasons people abandon goals: either losing hope in their capability to eventually succeed or feeling overwhelmed by the necessary effort and instead seeking easier short-term gratification. Both barriers relate to mindset. The growth perspective celebrates small gains as an indication that we are slowly expanding our potential, even if the ultimate goal remains distant. It also prioritizes consistent effort itself rather than any singular benchmark. Progress proceeds through constant pursuit.

Cultivating Growth Mindset

We can strengthen our thinking by being aware of negative beliefs that hold us back and choosing to see things in a more positive light instead. Here are some strategies that can help with that:

- **Recognize fixed mindset traps**: Notice negative self-talk focused on static traits or the shrinking effort required for growth. These negative influences try to tell you that your worth, talent, and capacity peak at some predetermined limit. Know that your potential is without limits.

- **Identify current mindsets**: Which fields like artistry, athletics, or academics present fixed ideas that natural talent alone is what determines capability? Consider the opposite message. Ability grows through practice. Skills develop over time. We are always deepening our self-knowledge.

- **Embrace challenges**: Rather than viewing discomfort as an indication we lack the necessary skill, reframe difficulty as a signal we have entered the optimal zone for significant learning. Lean constructively into the edges of competence. Growth lives outside of comfort zones.

- **Don't fear failure**: Setbacks offer invaluable feedback, revealing specific areas that need targeted strengthening. Each stumble holds inherent educational value about important next steps forward. Framing falls as fertilizer pushes our growth.

- **Value effort**: Consistency builds on itself—small daily progress adds up to extraordinary gains over time. Focus on the process itself, not just distant goals. What action can you thoughtfully commit to now without attaching it to specific outcomes?

- **Continue learning**: Adopt a student mindset, regardless of your life stage. Wisdom teaches us that a cup already full of its contents cannot receive fresh nectar. Empty cups thirstily welcome new liquids. Remain open and curious.

- **Cultivate persistence**: Mental fortitude correlates with a higher tolerance for uncertainty and discomfort. Practice moving toward growth zones at the edge of current competence. Encourage your grit. Skillfully manage frustration.

- **Seek constructive feedback**: Ask mentors and peers for guidance, identifying both strengths and developmental areas requiring focused practice to reach elevated performance. Feedback fuels improvement.

- **Model others' growth**: Notice those who have cultivated talents through long-term, dedicated effort. Recall that masters were once beginners themselves. Allow such examples to expand your beliefs about human potential.

- **Highlight improvements**: Journal about or proudly discuss with a trusted friend the growth you achieve in various areas of life. Perhaps creativity, social skills, career, health, or relationships. Even small gains deserve celebration.

The way we see ourselves has a lot to do with the things we tell ourselves all the time. When we believe we can learn and grow over time rather than think our talents are fixed, it helps us be more resilient even when facing big obstacles. Your brain is amazing; it can do great things if you encourage it with positive thoughts instead of putting yourself down.

Believe in your potential and ability to take on challenges through effort. Your thoughts shape your brain, so aim high!

Part 3:

Amplifying Resilience Through Social Bonds and Positive Habits

Part 2

Amplifying Resilience Thought

Social Bonds and Creative Habits

Chapter 6:
The Circle of Strength—Harnessing Social Support in Building Resilience

The year 2020 threw us for a loop! That new coronavirus showed up out of nowhere, and before we knew it, everything was changing. Families had to hunker down at home instead of going out, offices closed up shop, hospitals got overloaded quickly, and economies that seemed fine suddenly tanked. Too many people even lost their lives. What a crazy upheaval! Yet the people who handled all the chaos and uncertainty best usually had something helping them: staying in close touch with others. Even with so much fear about what was to come, consistent connections with friends and family helped ease the anxiety over cloudy horizons.

Abuelas in Ecuador, Italy, and beyond leaned out windows, sharing laughter, home-cooked meals, and amateur trumpet concerts with neighbors. Friends scattered across quarantining countries organized virtual game nights to spark joy and bond while isolated in their respective flats. Multigenerational families embraced simple pleasures like baking favorite recipes together or sharing stories from ancestors who survived wars, epidemics, and depressions decades prior—finding courage in recounted tales of resilience.

Such collective closeness served as a potent balm, easing helplessness against an invisible, unpredictable enemy. Humans thrive in a heartwarming community, especially amid overwhelming trials. While lonely souls certainly can demonstrate inspiring resilience, most discover profound purpose by courageously walking together with others toward a shared vision of possibility. As the African proverb reminds us, "If you want to travel fast, go alone. But if you want to travel far, go together." When facing sizable adversity, the load feels lighter when carried in compassionate company.

As individuals, we each embody a restricted capacity to dismantle systemic injustice, heal a community at odds with one another, restore harmony across factions, be open to hearing opposing views, or resolve any large problem alone. Yet, communities that stay together hold promise for mending divides by appealing to universal longings for love, trust, respect, and stability that most strongly desire but feel lacking.

With echo chambers stopping honest discourse and social technology, unfortunately, escalating conflict, we must re-learn relational abilities that foster goodwill. How do we proactively build resilient circles fortified to withstand differences of opinion yet anchored securely enough in shared humanity and hope to bridge the communication gaps haunting society?

Cultivating community resilience first requires intentional self-mastery practices that strengthen individual stability while also enhancing social skills that enable cooperative alliances. In isolation, we remain vulnerable, reeds bowing wherever the winds of influence blow strongest. But bundled together, we bond into sturdy and supportive forests.

We each hold responsibility for either depleting collective morale or uplifting spirits. By strengthening resilient communication and thinking before entering public discourse, our exchanges prove more fruitful in finding common ground.

When there's so much conflict everywhere, it's easy to feel like we need to stand up for ourselves and fight back against what we see as unfair or unkind. Some people think the answer is to completely ignore other points of view. However, many influential leaders of the past who promoted peace—like Jesus, Mahatma Gandhi, and Dr. Martin Luther King—showed us a better way. They dealt with problems directly and bravely while also staying calm and kind. Instead of reacting angrily or shutting others out, they engaged in disagreements in a spirit of understanding. We can do the same. When tensions rise, we don't have to make things worse; we can make them better. By keeping an open heart and respecting the truth on all sides, positive solutions are possible. All it takes is willing, thoughtful people coming together regularly to learn from each other and take constructive action. Small groups like that can spark big improvements, as long as the focus stays on personal and social improvement rather than personal attacks. Working this way, we have a real chance at progress.

As you read the forthcoming pages, consider what personal shifts support resilience for yourself and your community. How might you proactively uplift your immediate circles toward hope and help establish linkages between groups? During an era of uncertainty, isolation only compounds fear and weakness. But through interconnected resilience, we strengthen reserves of goodwill and moral strength, supporting a just society where all might thrive. The first steps begin with inner work that ripples outward.

The Power of We: Social Connections in Resilience Building

The year 2020 unleashed a storm of adversity unlike most living generations have endured before—an invisible pathogen seeding viral chaos and claiming millions of lives and livelihoods practically overnight. Yet even as poisonous anxiety hung heavy, those weathering the crisis with greater resilience often shared a protective buffer: a consistent connection.

Understanding Social Connections

Humans thrive through community. Our species survives due to interdependence and the collective potential of layered relationships meeting physical and emotional needs. Human connections are the mental, emotional, and physical bonds linking us to others in varying degrees of closeness.

This bonding manifests in varied forms including:

- **Friendships**: showing up for peers consistently.
- **Family ties**: unconditional belonging.
- **Romantic partnerships**: intimate vulnerability.
- **Community groups**: sharing values and experiences.
- **Online interactions**: digital support.

- **Service commitments**: contribution bonds.

Even just a quick, friendly interaction with someone we don't know can remind us that we're all in this together. A smile or kind word from a stranger has a way of lifting our spirits. Our close friends and family who've been there for the long haul are especially important; they're the safe place we can turn to when life gets hard. We know we have people to open up to about our struggles who will support us through it all and help us rebuild.

Having that strong network of support makes it a bit easier to get through tough times. Sometimes coming out the other side of difficulties helps us help others deal with their storms one day. The friends who helped carry us might need us in return. So, by sharing each other's burdens, over time our community can take hardship and turn it into the power to ease suffering for many. Connecting with each other is what sees people through to better days.

Social Connections Build Resilience

During seasons of trauma, relationships literally buffer our basic survival mechanisms. The calming act of hugging a trusted friend lowers blood pressure, heart rate, and anxiety. Close bonds drive up feel-good neurotransmitters like oxytocin and serotonin, alleviating depressive tendencies. Chronic isolation, conversely, weakens immune function and accelerates disease pathways (Cuffari, 2023).

Individuals enjoying meaningful communal connections consistently demonstrate heightened resilience and longevity compared to those lacking social support, however independent in their personalities (Hetherington, 2023). Our connections provide ballast, hedging against hardship's hazards.

Benefits of Strong Social Ties

Cultivating communities pays exponential dividends, strengthening overall well-being through:

- **Boosted mental health**: By sharing troubles and celebrating wins with trusted allies, we ease burdened thoughts, gain encouragement, and feel understood, rather than bottling frustrations alone. Confidants help reframe situations constructively.

- **Increased longevity**: Research reveals those surrounded by positive social circles live longer on average while also exhibiting decreased risk for diseases like heart disease, stroke, and dementia compared to isolated peers (Harvard College, 2019). Humans thrive when cherished.

- **Improved quality of living**: Community involvement fosters a greater sense of meaning and self-efficacy. Contributing our skills makes life feel purposeful. Receiving loving receptivity in return builds self-worth. We lift each other higher.

- **Decreased risk of suicide**: Suicidal individuals who list few accessible social supports are more likely to act negatively during crises, whereas those surrounded by non-judgmental ears walk forward with hope, meaning, and grit to endure momentary setbacks.

Not all relationships are good for your mental health. Some connections might be harmful if they involve hostility or abuse. These kinds of draining relationships can make vulnerable people feel even more alone and promote unhealthy habits. Whether the people in your life tend to make you feel better or worse is something you should consider. Spending time with caring friends and family is crucial for helping each person deal with life's challenges. When you surround yourself with a community that supports you, it provides an emotional support system, so you feel less shaken by hardships. You bounce back more quickly from tough times because you have people you can count on.

During an era of uncertainty and social distancing, outreach bridging divides proves more important than ever. A kind word, compassionate deed, or genuine smile even behind masked faces affirms shared humanity present despite any surface differences. Familiar gathering places closed overnight during early pandemic waves, yet resilient communities cultivated connection creatively through new mediums as village life migrated to the digital space.

What proactive steps will you take today to extend warmth to another isolated soul? Your small act multiplied by consistent effort seeds the very culture our hearts crave—emphasizing people over problems. Together, through empathy and equity, we fortify reserves of goodwill and moral strength, supporting a society where all might thrive. Our collective resilience awaits cooperative care.

Nurturing Bonds

Relationships serve as anchors securing us during storms and sails catching wind to accelerate toward hope. Yet that magical spell of bonding individuals requires skillful nurturing through self-knowledge, consistent care, and communicating even when conflicts naturally arise. By planting seeds of empathy and actively cultivating compassion, our most significant connections flourish for years while weathering occasional droughts.

Building Supportive Relationships

Creating uplifting relationships with loved ones, friends, family, and the community requires one to:

- **Know yourself**: Grow clearer on your values, communication style, emotional needs, past relational patterns, and vision for an ideal healthy relationship, dynamic, or friendship. Self-awareness allows for clearly articulating desires to others.

- **Develop people skills**: Practice listening fully without interrupting, validate others' experiences naturally, initiate enjoyable conversations, collaborate on conflict resolution, and show consistent care through involvement. These abilities deepen over time through concerted effort.

- **Respect and appreciation**: Assume positive intent when misunderstandings occur. Catch yourself complaining excessively or critically nitpicking. Instead, intentionally praise and give attention to loved ones' shining qualities and express sincere gratitude often. We see what we spotlight.

- **Accept and celebrate differences**: Variety across personalities and cultural upbringings contributes richness to relationships. Discuss variances in preferences compassionately without insisting on a strict or uniform way of being. Conflict only arises when one forces the other to change rather than giving space for individual expression. Live and let live.

- **Practice effective communication**: Speak clearly, matching volume, vocabulary, and speed to the circumstances and listener, while encouraging feedback. Assert needs and boundaries kindly, without aggression. Listen fully before thoughtfully responding. Master both articulate expression and receptive understanding.

- **Spend quality time**: Prioritize regular one-on-one interaction free of distractions, building trust through shared activities, accountability discussions, collaborative planning, inside jokes, and heartfelt dialogue conveying care.

- **Develop shared interests**: Bond over mutually enjoyable hobbies, such as exploring nature, creating art, playing games, traveling, volunteering together, attending live events, researching captivating topics, and so on. Common passions unite.

- **Be dependable**: When promising to connect at set times, follow through consistently. Avoid canceling without a legitimate reason and without warning others impacted. Show up fully present when together. Reliability builds security knowing you remain unwavering in their corner.

Maintaining Supportive Relationships

Keeping relationships thriving over the years requires an ongoing commitment to growth and grace:

- **Put in the work**: Don't assume bonds will deepen without active investment. Make deposits of care by creating enjoyable experiences, sending reminders that you are thinking of them, verbally affirming strengths, and maintaining physical and emotional availability without overextending yourself.

- **Set and respect boundaries**: Communicate clearly what supports make you feel most loved and respected. If scheduling focused friend time weekly nourishes your soul, assert that need kindly. Reciprocate respecting the other's declared requirements. Find a compromise that aligns both parties when possible.

- **Talk and listen well**: Foster open, non-defensive dialogue addressing issues promptly before tension escalates unhealthy resentment over unspoken grievances. Seek mutual understanding. Provide a safe space for each individual's authentic expression and empathic reception.

- **Give affection and appreciation**: Love manifests a universal language of acknowledging another's precious presence through gifts matching their preference—quality time, physical touch, encouraging words, helpful acts of service, or other personal pleasures. Show them your essence through thoughtful showings of affection.

- **Prioritize the relationship**: Protect bonds from weakening by scheduling uninterrupted couple or best friend time, safeguarding space for reconnection amid busy individual demands. Routine togetherness renews fondness.

- **Exercise flexibility**: Embrace the inevitable change accompanying seasons of life, from having kids to switching careers or moving across town, interfering with previous comfortable routines. Adjust attitudes before resenting external shifts out of your control. What matters most remains a caring company.

- **Argue fairly**: Arguments emerge in even healthy bonds. Handle conflict constructively by identifying the true root issues respectfully, without character assassination. Take space if needed before reengaging with gentler language, seeking compromise. Move on fully later.

- **Give and receive support**: Practice being vulnerable, sharing personal struggles, and offering empathic space should the other confide in you their emotional pains or ask for practical help. Mutual consolation cements intimacy durably, enduring all weathers.

Like any living organism, relationships evolve beyond initial bloom, carrying undercurrents of difficulty or delight through longevity. By planting seeds of self-knowledge, communicating clearly, and keeping care as the consistent priority fertilizing fondness, connections thrive, securing us through inevitable storms and reveling in life's joy. Nurture your tribes well.

The Role of Communication in Relationships

Legend tells of two estranged brothers, once inseparable as children, now avoiding family holidays to dodge tense reunions, recalling old grudges. Over the years apart, with minimal communication, each crafted his own self-preserving narrative. "He always claimed Mom's affection and ignored my interests and needs. His arrogance is unbearable," fumed one brother. The other recounts differently: "I constantly tried engaging him as a kid. He repaid my efforts by calling me annoying. Now he coldly pretends I don't exist."

Their thorny relationship history and current silence fuel easy offense, mistrust, and exhaustion when inevitably gathering at their parents' 50th-anniversary party. Rather than directly discussing old wounds, the brothers evade and exchange mere cursory greetings before separating across the house. Another chance at reconciliation slips by. Pain continues to grow from assumptions filling the communication gap.

Our closest relationships often shape foundational feelings about self-worth, trust, and hope. Yet without skillful relating habits, bonds may fray from misunderstandings, unrealistic expectations, and pent-up frustrations, obscuring a partner's or friend's humanity behind our own narrow hurt. Let's discuss how communication fosters connection.

Communication Fuels Connection

Effective communication weaves into the very fabric of relationships, cementing them as bonds that stand the test of time and conflict. Speaking honestly and listening generously prevents common pitfalls like resentment, distrust, and chronic frustration threatening fondness. Core skills include:

- fostering safety through vulnerable sharing.

- accurately conveying our lived experience.

- receptive understanding when roles are reversed.

Relationships relying primarily on assumptions rather than gentle communication often deteriorate as injured parties construct imagined narratives, feeling convincing but lacking grounding in reality. Routinely engaging in open, thoughtful dialogue provides necessary support during inevitable challenges.

How exactly does communication nourish relationships and foster resilience even amid conflict?

- **Builds trust**: Consistent transparency around needs, hurts, or hopes prevent spiraling anxiety from making up stories when silence breeds uncertainty. Honest expression builds faith; the other person remains relatable, reliable, and caring despite ups and downs.

- **Defuses misunderstandings**: We often underestimate how differently two people register the same event, omitting pivotal context clues from our internal replay. Clarifying intended meanings dispels inaccurate interpretations, protecting bonds and preventing the wrong conclusion from being reached.

- **Develops mutual respect**: Speaking plainly about boundaries and listening earnestly when receiving another's builds empathy and insight. This shows that even loved ones see life through alternate lenses, prioritizing certain preferences, reactions, or values subjectively. We broaden our worldviews by entering alternate realities.

- **Prevents hurtful guesswork**: Rather than imagining how friends or family might act during the confusion and ascribing false motives needlessly, brave inquiry extracts answers directly from the source. Despite discomfort approaching conflicts, clarity alleviates invented worries without concrete data.

- **Boosts positive sentiment**: Both expressing appreciation and thoughtful praise or simply conveying "I love and care for you" transcend surface moods, reconnecting partners to fond foundations. Warm attention exchanges release pleasurable neurochemicals!

- **Strengthens relationship ties**: Asking engaging questions about growth edges sparks meaningful dialogue. Playfully bantering inside jokes invites laughter. Recalling cherished memories and dreaming together revives intimacy. The act of sharing meaningfully weaves sturdy relational threads over decades if consistently practiced.

- **Opens new possibilities**: Curiosity fertilizes growth! What long-held dreams, recent epiphanies, or brewing fears occupy your best friend's mind today? You will never know unless your curious and exploratory words wrap this beloved soul with affirming attention. Such gifts enable more authentic relationships.

- **Reduces toxic rumination**: Voicing frustrations bothering us alleviates corrosive thoughts, repeating on a loop when left unspoken. Once aired, troubles feel lighter and we clear bandwidth, focusing positively on shared visions rather than stewing silently about impediments.

- **Cultivates deeper intimacy**: Vulnerability remains reciprocal. Offering kind space when others unveil their layered complexity nurtures an instinctual trust to also reveal our hidden selves. Soulful communion requires risk to unfold fully. What revelations await among known faces made unfamiliar by long-withheld perspectives?

- **Defuses destructive conflict**: Nipping misunderstandings promptly preserves goodwill before issues snowball into explosive altercations or lingering cold wars. Skillfully surfacing tensions calmly with "I" language breathes connection into quarrels by underscoring mutual commitment and surviving turmoil.

Just as oil lubricates mechanical parts moving cooperatively, consistent communication ensures relationships flow smoothly together toward shared dreams, rather than away from each other into isolation. We must champion dialogue, courageously shepherding bonds from fragility to deep resilience, ready to withstand gathering storms.

Strategies for Effective Communication and Seeking Help

Legend tells of two respected tribal elders, known as astute advisors, who each provided counsel widely on personal dilemmas or guidance in navigating group disputes. Villagers remark on their uncannily accurate insights into misunderstandings and gifts for awakening warmth between bitterly feuding families. What wisdom has forged such discernment and skill for reconciliation?

The first elder begins her meditative morning ritual, envisioning each community member glowing with inner brilliance as a vessel of the ancestral stream. "Help me see through surface masks today to know your true essence," she whispers, nodding respectfully toward the rising sun.

The second elder simply listens. For hours on end, he sits, welcoming seekers to unburden their hearts without interruption. Through patient silence, torrents of truths too long dammed flood forth. "In listening deeply, wounded spirits often trace confusion back to their core needs," observes the sage, nodding in rhythm to their words.

Effective communication weaves relationships into sturdy tapestries stronger than individual threads alone. While mastering key skills takes commitment, subtle shifts reap exponential dividends. Consider adopting these proven techniques for elevating connections.

Hone Communication Capacity

Compassionate communication means accurately expressing our inner world while receptively entering another's without confusion. Essentials include:

- **Listen actively**: Give complete attention to the speaker without interrupting. Maintain eye contact and an open posture. Reflect on key points to confirm shared understanding. Show interest by asking thoughtful questions before respectfully voicing any differing views non-defensively.

- **Focus on one topic**: Reduce confusion by addressing one situation or issue at a time. Once a resolution is reached regarding the initial subject, the partner should summarize the agreements before carefully broaching another nuanced conversation requiring similarly undivided bandwidth.

- **Adapt to audiences**: Adjust vocabulary, speed, examples, and volume, aligning the message with cultural familiarity, education levels, learning styles, language fluency, or other needs of those listening. Create optimal conditions for comprehension.

- **Consider body language**: Be aware of and adapt facial expressions, hand motions, posture, and proximity respectfully when speaking or listening. Nonverbal cues significantly color verbal content, conveying emotions subtly. Ensure harmony between gestures and words.

- **Check for clarity**: Seeking reflective feedback safeguards against assuming messages are transmitted clearly. Kindly verify what ideas others heard rather than presuming to prevent communication breakdowns that erode relationships over time. Misunderstandings often loom quietly.

- **Speak concisely**: Precise expression demonstrates respect for listeners' time and attention spans. Prepare succinct yet descriptive phrasing, emphasizing the essence. Lead with the primary point or request before elaborating on relevant details when useful.

- **Take purposeful notes**: Write down key topics discussed, commitments made, insights gained, and follow-up questions to revisit later during complex conversations. These scribbles jog clarity and accountability after interactions conclude.

- **Consider calling**: While convenient for rapid response, text or email communication risks misinterpretation. They lack vocal tone and instant feedback to explain intended meanings should any confusion arise. During tense situations especially, choose synchronous mediums permitting real-time exchange.

- **Think before speaking**: Pause before reacting to emotionally charged content, allowing the initial wave to settle. Then consciously reflect on both context and the ideal outcome before forming a thoughtful, level-headed response or consciously deciding not to engage further.

- **Respect all equally**: Honor each person's inherent worth by listening patiently without prejudice when opinions differ from your own experiences. Seek shared truth, upholding dignity. Judging or belittling breeds defensiveness rather than mutual understanding.

- **Expand emotional intelligence**: Grow self-awareness around personal triggers, tendencies when overwhelmed, and destructive communication habits. Notice these arising and adapt accordingly. Manage frustration wisely.

- **Develop workplace communication norms**: Establish team communication expectations and preferred channels that suit workflows. Model these consistently, especially regarding meeting etiquette and email correspondence. Nip any confusion promptly.

- **Foster organizational belonging**: Facilitate rapport and psychological safety among colleagues through team-building activities, recognizing achievements publicly, and maintaining open-door policies welcoming idea exchange. Together, everyone achieves more!

While mastering communication requires lifelong practice, small improvements reap exponential progress. What skill seems within reach but promises huge relationship rewards with a bit more mindfulness today?

Chapter 7:
Daily Doses of Resilience—Habits That Bolster Your Bounce-Back Ability

Legend tells of two young maple trees sprouting side-by-side in spring, both stretching leafy arms skyward to soak up the first rains after winter's thaw. As balmy breezes shift to summer's oppressive humidity, the first tree begins to die, while the second continues to flourish, seemingly impervious to the unrelenting heat.

"What's your secret?" asks the faded maple, exhausted from unsuccessfully battling the elements.

"Simple. I dig deep each dawn, strengthening my roots before dancing with seasonal change. By anchoring internally first, I freely move when storms inevitably arrive," beams the vibrant tree, still swaying gracefully despite the burning sunshine.

The seedlings illustrate that individual physiques can variously determine natural resilience reserves, over which we hold no control. Yet tending to daily habits and strengthening foundational well-being proves vital for surviving sudden environmental shocks.

In chaos theory, scientists closely study complex systems, demonstrating that a butterfly flapping its wings in the Amazon significantly alters weather patterns as far as Bangladesh months later through a cascading effect over time and distance (Oestreicher, 2007). So too can small, consistent actions that seed mental and physical health support stabilize our psyches for withstanding turbulent times.

The small practices with the wide impact that this chapter addresses include building resilient psychological viewpoints that allow for flexibility when accustomed systems are uprooted and enhancing resilience via self-care and community.

Self-care serves as the bedrock for individual resilience, strengthening the energy needed to support others during crises. Essentials include:

- **Mindset matters**: Our lens colors reality. Adopt empowering narratives that reinforce the capability to eventually overcome challenges through strategic persistence. Acknowledge all progress made.

- **Move your body**: Regular movement energizes, reduces anxiety and depression, and buffers immune function, protecting overall wellness during chaotic periods inhospitable to health.

- **Nurture nature**: Spend time immersed in natural settings, promoting cognitive restoration from draining demands. Nature's inherent peace restores balance when turmoil surrounds us.

- **Fuel well**: Energy, moods, and focus improve when eating whole, nutritious foods. Refined sugars and complex carbs boost resilience. Stay hydrated and nourished, and trim cravings with clean fuel.

- **Sleep deeply**: Effective rest makes one feel refreshed, focused, and flexible at the start of the day, key for addressing complex situations. Protect sleep quality by keeping technology out of bedrooms.

- **Cultivate community wellness**: Individual health depends on collective health. Creating cultures of trust, inclusion, and care where all feel valued strengthens group morale to cooperatively withstand adversity.

- **Foster workplace resilience**: Organizational resilience requires addressing wellness systemically through policies that nurture stability.

- **Flexible scheduling**: Accommodate caregiving demands and disability needs with options like flextime, condensed schedules, or remote work balanced against business requirements.

- **Boundaries**: Discourage emailing after hours and excessively working through lunch or days off. Model utilizing paid time off for whole health.

- **Self-care training**: Host workshops teaching stress management, nutrition, or movement breaks. Consider separating money toward wellness expenses like gym memberships or meditation apps.

- **Trauma training**: Educate leadership on common psychological responses to collective disasters like pandemics so they can sensitively support staff through grief and stress.

- **Social support**: Facilitate informal peer support groups for counseling, empathy, and accountability toward achieving shared objectives.

Let's continue exploring small tips, designing wide doors for societies where all people might access tools to not only survive but even thrive through trouble. Just as barnacles accumulate slowly on ship hulls navigating rough seas, so too must we actively care for emotional vessels vulnerable to dread when battered by waves of worry. I wish you fair winds and calm waters, resilient ones!

Habits of Steel

Our actions over time shape who we are. Therefore, excellence is a habit rather than an act, as noted by the philosopher Will Durant. An estimated 40% of our daily actions unfold habitually without conscious thought, freeing bandwidth for novel duties (Linder et al., 2021). Habits effectively develop the muscle memory to navigate regular routines seamlessly.

The Power of Habits

Habits evolve organically through the consistent repetition of behaviors our minds and bodies find efficient. Triggered by familiar cues like arriving home or an alarm sounding, we operate on autopilot, reaching for sneakers to go jogging or catching up on social media without a thought.

Such engrained ritualistic tendencies heavily influence responses when daily impulses drastically shift unexpectedly, like relationships ending, careers upending, disasters striking, or dreams dying. Those lacking resilient-minded habits often reactively crumble, while individuals grounded in persistent routines capitalize on inherent mental strength to adapt constructively.

Resilience Relies on Habits

Resilience indicates the capacity to recover in the face of adversity—to flex rather than fracture when external forces apply pressure. Bouncing back requires accessing internal resources and healthy coping outlets to process difficulty, identify options, determine a strategic response, emotionally re-stabilize after disruptions, and ultimately reinforce persistence for future storms.

Routines centering on self-care, social support, optimistic perspectives, and organization systems strengthen resilience through repetition, like casting psychological safety nets and anticipating imbalance. Fitness habits create physical stability and mental balance to address problems proactively. The instinctual tendency to lean on learned behaviors for support through uncharted chaos underscores the value of consciously curating habits aligned with resilience.

Anecdote About How Habits Build Resilience

Consider motivational speaker Gerhard Le Roux, who transformed his mindset and thus his life trajectory by harnessing the power of small habits—first while imprisoned, then through rebuilding post-release.

Despite childhood poverty and no secondary education, Gerhard became an entrepreneur and loving family man before losing everything over fraud charges. After divorce and strained relationships, he found himself jailed with few prospects in sight. Though the situation appeared hopeless, Gerhard planted seeds of promise through life-affirming routines completed despite being imprisoned and in distress.

He nurtured gratitude and optimism. He exercised vigorously rather than staying in depression. He prayed, meditated, and wrote self-affirmations. He devoured empowering books and resources, furthering self-education. Just as rock climbers carefully select footfalls up sheer mountainsides, so too can we elevate existence foothold by foothold through purposeful habits, even when lacking wider control over realities.

Upon exiting prison, still left with excessive debt, Gerhard continued positive rituals. Now additionally working multiple jobs, strictly budgeting, and networking strategic connections for his speaking career, he eventually achieved remarkable stability and success. Now he shares a message of responsibility and proactivity, birthing resilience. His story underscores that while we cannot control all external variables, our internal habits impact responses.

Practical Habits for Building Resilience

Let Gerhard's incredible demonstration of resilience inspire your habit formation. How might small actions seed incredible growth? Consider adopting these practices:

- **Prioritize restorative sleep**: Protect sleep sanctity from digital disruptions. Realigning rhythms takes time but restores processing capacity, supporting resilient perspectives.

- **Exercise more**: Any movement—walking, dancing, strengthening muscles, or sports—releases feel-good endorphins that sustain emotional balance and physical health when trials arise.

- **Seek social support**: Connect often with uplifting individuals who compassionately listen, offer perspective, and cheer on progress. Shared burdens feel lighter.

- **Accept help without shame**: We all occasionally struggle. Allow trusted allies to lift you rather than hiding in isolation, exhausting limited emotional bandwidth already depleted by hardship. Release pride and embrace grace.

- **Avoid self-blame**: When reevaluating missteps, speak to yourself as a trusted advisor might respectfully highlight strengths, opportunities, and realistic next steps.

- **Make peace with the past**: Pain cannot be changed. Yet holding grudges against people or life for lost dreams or perceived injustice occupies precious mental space, better focused on creating hope.

- **Welcome change as an opportunity**: Flexibly flowing with new seasons, while uncomfortable initially, fosters growth. What possibilities shine amid uncertainty? The cocoon must shatter for wings to grace the skies.

While life offers no guarantees, consciously developing habits and building mental muscle empowers resilience to face difficulties inevitable for butterflies and humans alike. What small practices might you adopt today? Small roots are stabilizing mighty oaks through coming storms.

Self-Care: Your Path to Personal Wellness

Self-care refers to the daily practices and rituals we deliberately choose to nourish our whole selves—body, mind, and spirit. The many dimensions of health are dependent on one another, so attending to emotional needs proves just as important as eating nutritious foods, moving the physical form, stimulating creativity, and resting deeply.

At its core, self-care means strategically adjusting daily activities to align with your values and needs rather than operating on autopilot, listening to external demands alone. It requires reflection and honestly assessing, "What practices would support my best self?" Then self-care involves adopting supportive habits and prioritizing wellness despite competing responsibilities. Think of it as decentralized healthcare beginning from within rather than waiting reactively when already burned out by life's relentless responsibilities.

Embracing self-compassion helps silence that nagging inner critic questioning whether we deserve nourishing activities when so much human suffering exists in the world. How can people justify indulgent self-care? Yet pouring from an empty cup simply rinses our capacity to uplift anyone at all! Self-care permits consistently showing up as our best selves wherever needed most.

Self-Care Promotes Holistic Wellness

Attending to self-care nourishes well-being across connected dimensions:

- physical health through nutrition, movement, and rest
- mental health via mindfulness, therapy, and creative flow
- emotional health by processing feelings
- spiritual health through meaning and connection
- environmental health in our living and working spaces
- financial health by aligning career, spending, and values
- social health in our relationships
- and career health, discussing career fit

Taking care of your own needs is important for your overall health and strength. Setting and maintaining your own needs comes first and benefits your physical, mental, and emotional wellness. It's kind of like different colored strings that together form a sturdy net. The net protects you during tough personal times and also during rough patches affecting the whole community. Making yourself feel good inside and out through things like relaxation, healthy habits, and self-compassion weaves everything together to create a solid support system.

Self-Care Builds Resilience

During the pandemic, healthcare providers worldwide reported an alarming 25% increase in anxiety and depression worldwide (World

Health Organization, 2022). However, those intentionally pausing for self-care proved less depleted long-term.

Research confirms the link between self-care and resilience across populations. A 2022 study among palliative teams showed mindful self-care practices correlated to resilience against pandemic-related burnout (Garcia et al., 2022). Self-care buffered work-life impairment and boosted workplace thriving.

Similarly, breast cancer patients coping resiliently developed self-care habits like light exercise, stress reduction, and maintaining social ties, ultimately rating their quality of life higher despite their devastating diagnosis (Ristevska-Dimitrovska et al., 2015). Psychologists determine that engaging in self-care mediates resilience and well-being, exponentially empowering us to withstand adversity.

Individual well-being and collective resilience intertwine. Each small act of self-care that benefits emotional reserves communicates our inherent worth, while also seeding a culture that compels organizations and communities to defend space for nourishing humanity. The radical act of caring first for ourselves ripples outward in our steadfast refusal to reduce people into machines, always expected to function regardless of soulful needs.

Healing begins as an inside job. How will you choose to nourish your overall well-being today? Your commitment sparks a chain reaction, reminding others that their whole humanity matters too, even under pressing conditions. A new norm elevating self-care plants resilient seeds, uplifting society.

Self-Care Tips

Legend tells of a thriving garden, abundantly yielding healing herbs and vibrant vegetables year after year and season after season while neighboring plots slowly died. Curious neighbors asked the magical gardener how her emerald oasis flourished even amid oppressive weather.

"I care evenly for the interconnected elements, so foundational roots spread deeply, sturdy stems reach toward light, and ripe fruit feeds each element in interdependence," replied the nurturing village herbalist, scattering homegrown compost and ensuring yet another fruitful harvest.

Her wisdom reminds us that self-care involves attending to multiple dimensions of our being through nurturing practices, fostering holistic wellness as the surest path to personal resilience. Consider weaving these ideas into your daily life.

Physical Self-Care

The body serves as a precious vehicle for transporting the mind and spirit. Core maintenance helps optimize functioning during all seasons.

- **Prioritize restorative sleep**: Protect sleep consistently without digital disruptions, realigning natural rhythms. Proper restoration requires downtime-integrating experiences that minimize anxiety and depression.

- **Incorporate balanced nutrition**: Energy, moods, and focus improve by eating whole, nutritious foods. Refined sugars and complex carbs boost resilience. Stay hydrated and reduce inflammation through antioxidants.

- **Make time for movement**: Any physical activity releases feel-good endorphins and maintains healthy immunity and focus. Walk, stretch, dance, play sports—whatever you enjoy! Start small, yet make it routine.

- **Modulate stimulant intake**: Limit caffeine, alcohol, or excessive media usage that overstimulates delicate nervous systems, interrupts sleep, and depletes emotional reserves needed to weather storms. Everything is in moderation.

Emotional Self-Care

Identifying, expressing, and adapting feelings prevents repression from boiling over destructively. Emotional fitness allows for appropriately channeling anger, disappointment, or grief when adversity strikes. Essentials include:

- **Know your vulnerabilities**: Pinpoint tendencies like trauma triggers, negative thought loops, or poor boundaries that could permit emotional hijacking. Define the needed conditions for supporting security.

- **Engage socially with supportive people**: Connect regularly with trusted individuals who compassionately listen, offer perspective, and cheer progress. Shared burdens feel lighter. Choose your company carefully.

- **Prepare ahead of time to avoid feeling overwhelmed**: Monitor emotional capacity to identify rising tension early. Temporarily reduce commitments, preventing overload. Allow for processing time and support. Say no without guilt.

- **Set loving limits**: Communicate needs and boundaries kindly yet firmly. Be specific about what nourishes your spirit and what you find depleting. Protect your energy.

- **Learn relaxation skills**: Practice calming nerves and adjusting big feelings by breathing deeply, moving thoughtfully, writing feelings out, praying, or creating art. Consider counseling that explores childhood patterns that are still subconsciously triggered.

- **Reestablish predictable routines**: Much chaos remains beyond our control; embrace what is while accepting limitations. But restore personal order within each new normal through consistent morning rituals, life administration systems, reasonable to-do lists, and early bedtimes.

- **Listen to uplifting music and podcasts**: Create playlists that build positivity. Sing aloud or dance freely. Find speakers that make you hopeful. Music significantly impacts moods, motivation, and mindset. Use its power wisely.

Social Self-Care

Humans thrive in a healthy community. Invest in fulfilling relationships.

- **Stay alert to withdrawal urges**: Note tendencies to isolate when overwhelmed, which further aggravates stress. Lean into loved ones offering uplifting perspectives. If spirits feel chronically low, seek counseling support groups.

- **Infuse social engagements**: Search for therapists who can help make your recovery a more social process by reviewing professional certification bodies in your area. *MeetMe* provides a space where you can meet and chat with new people who share your interest in accountable progress check-ins, leisurely fun, and purposeful causes. Schedule video calls, outdoor meetups, and recreation time if they are unavailable in person during the chaos.

- **Give and request encouragement**: You can share small victories or funny stories with your friends and family. You can use *Facebook* stories, *Instagram*, *WhatsApp* stories, and *TikTok* if you are on social media. If you're not on social media you can still share with your friends and family in person! Celebrate someone else's wins. Ask trusted allies for reassurance, reality checks, or help solving dilemmas. Offer the same graciously.

- **Laugh together**: Inject lightness. Play games involving creativity, movement, or humor. Laughter eases tense muscles and releases pleasure chemicals that benefit the body and soul.

- **Remember work relationships**: Foster professional bonds through collaborating, appreciating colleague efforts, and participating in office social events when possible. Align with company culture.

By proactively caring across the physical, mental, emotional, social, and vocational realms through simple daily practices, we compound stability and satisfaction exponentially. What small step can be taken today to improve overall health? You matter so very much to yourself, your loved ones, and our shared society! How shall we begin practicing resilient self-care?

Beat the Burnout: Effective Strategies for Stress Management

Like a kettle forgotten on the stove, once vibrant spirits slowly simmer to exhaustion if unrelenting demands persist without relief. In recent years, professionals across industries have reported skyrocketing stress and burnout threatening well-being in an age with an endless deluge of digital notifications and doom-scrolling news reels.

Burnout is a common problem among healthcare practitioners, mainly due to the high demands and stress involved in their work. A study discovered that around 50% of physicians in the United States suffer from burnout (Clark, 2021). Additionally, nurses and other healthcare workers also report experiencing high levels of burnout. Burnout is not just limited to the workforce, it can also affect students. A survey conducted by the American Psychological Association (APA) revealed that more than one-third of college students have experienced significant levels of psychological distress (Abrams, 2022). Academic pressure, high expectations, and balancing multiple responsibilities are major factors.

Recognizing the toll of unmanaged stress proves critical before it boils over and spills into chronic periods of overwhelming stress, sabotaging resilience.

What is Stress and Burnout?

Stress involves the body's natural activation response when demands outweigh available resources. Initially, chemical reactions prepare strength and speed for reacting to perceived danger, whether modern threats like work deadlines or evolutionarily life-threatening events like returning home to find your home destroyed.

According to a Gallup study, almost two-thirds of full-time employees in the United States experience burnout to some degree (Hemphill, 2022). The World Health Organization (WHO) has recognized burnout as an occupational phenomenon, emphasizing its impact on work environments.

Mild stress fuels productivity by meeting reasonable challenges. But as intensifying responsibilities turn up the burners for too long, excess heat gradually saps coping reserves until pipes rupture.

Prolonged states of overwhelming stress spark burnout—the state of emotional, mental, and physical exhaustion from chronic stress left untended for too long. Rather than an event, it evolves quietly, like veins marbled from plaque accumulation.

Impact on Health and Resilience

Unmanaged stress not only depletes energy day-to-day but built up can completely wipe out overall well-being. Intolerable demands frequently outstrip our coping capacity until our fuse eventually blows.

Studies link burnout to concerning health impacts like heart disease, diabetes, depression, anxiety, and early death (Koutsimani et al., 2019) (Kontoangelos et al., 2022). Constant distress also prevents resilience by draining mental strength and emotional flexibility, protecting against life's inevitable setbacks outside of work.

Like an exhausted hiker scaling endless mountainous terrain, individuals experiencing burnout feel emotionally, mentally, and physically drained by unrelenting demands exceeding available coping reserves. Gradually, one labored step follows another until they finally collapse, drained of motivation to continue uphill battles.

Yet long before that point of complete exhaustion, our minds and bodies communicate subtle symptoms indicative of built-up stress threatening overall health and resilience reserves if ignored. Tuning into these early warning signs allows for self-care strategies to prevent total depletion.

Physical Signals of Burnout

When facing unrelenting pressures, the body frequently issues fatigue, illness, or pain, signaling mounting distress.

- **Chronic exhaustion**: Difficulty arising each morning for duties that once felt easy, which indicates severe energy expenditure outpacing recovery. Listen to your cravings for extra sleep.

- **Falling immunity**: Recurring cold and flu symptoms or frequent infections hint at a compromised immune system, too stressed to fight internal illness.

- **Headaches and body aches**: When demands turn up the dial past their comfortable capacity, muscles tense, carrying the weight of responsibility, eventually straining into soreness, migraines, and back pain.

- **Appetite and sleep disruption**: Like an engine warning light, sudden weight fluctuations or insomnia communicate an imbalance somewhere in our operations. Determine where overload is occurring and adjust accordingly.

While pushing through mild discomfort enables handling temporary pressures, make note of bodily signals indicating too much pressure. Pain whispers at first, then shouts if ignored. Heed symptoms before they become serious.

Emotional Red Flags

In tandem with physical symptoms, psychological and emotional patterns offer clues that simmering stress may be spiraling into more harmful burnout if unaddressed.

- **Growing cynicism and misery**: Consistently dreading obligations and feeling tired of once enjoyable commitments hints that simmering strain has eaten away at former excitement for roles and is now feeling chronically overwhelming.

- **Detachment increases**: When even previously pleasurable pastimes or relationships no longer spark satisfaction, this withdrawal hints at profound fatigue, short-circuiting natural lightness.

- **Decreased motivation emerges**: If finding initiative toward regular responsibilities feels persistently burdensome, like trudging through thick mud, lowered motivation indicates simmering burnout. This burnout eats away at get-up-and-go determination, turning it into sighed resignation.

- **Pessimism traps loom**: Once evenly balanced perspectives and expectations shift into predominantly negative judgments, classifying all developments as somehow flawed or disappointing. Poisonous cynicism eats away at the optimism needed to fuel excellence and long-term satisfaction.

- **Plummeting self-efficacy**: As exhaustion sets in, confidence in the inability to handle quantities of work assignments drops significantly, replaced by creeping self-criticism and a comparative lack of mentality.

Reactive Behavior Changes Emerge

Accumulating internal stress sparks external behavioral changes like:

- **Withdrawing from commitments**: Isolation increases in proportion to the emotional resources available to engage meaningfully with others. Preserve energy for essentials.

- **Avoidance coping continues**: Excessive hours of mindlessly scrolling digital content or news often indicate an unconscious escape from complex realities, that ask more of us than we have to offer.

- **Procrastination spikes**: As duties feel increasingly oppressive, the tendency to perpetually defer unpleasant tasks intensifies while procrastination increases, making deadlines even more difficult.

- **Risky self-medicating**: Without healthy outlets balancing the load, substance misuse rates rise proportionately to distress levels as people attempt self-soothing urgency temporarily through quick means.

- **Blowing fuses finalize breakdown**: Irritability manifests through picking fights, blaming, complaining constantly, or lashing out as fumes run low. Tension seeks any exit for release.

Rather than soldiering through extreme stress dismissed as normal professional perseverance, acknowledge messages of malfunction. Just as vehicle dashboard lights indicate needing checkups, so too do minds and bodies communicate our personal need for urgent realignment through symptoms of burnout. Ensure you get needed nourishment immediately by setting healthy boundaries and requesting reasonable accommodation. Tomorrow's increased productivity relies on prioritizing sanity today.

Busting Stress and Burnout Myths

While experiencing burnout proves increasingly common in the modern era, outdated assumptions still paint exhaustion as a personal weakness rather than the result of dysfunctional systems overburdening us. Until we revise society's mindset on burnout, stigma persists, discouraging preventative self-care or transparent requests for reasonable accommodation. Let's demystify some of those harmful myths now.

Myth: Burnout Signals Weakness

Truth: Burnout develops when even healthy individuals continue under extreme, unrelenting stress. Redefine overwhelmed reactions as a sign of humanity, not inadequacy. We all have limits requiring respect.

Myth: Burnout Means You're Broken

Truth: Complete exhaustion is not inherently permanent. Balance can be restored through self-care and adjusting demands with enough recovery time and resources. Healing happens gradually. Be patient with the process.

Myth: Burnout Harms Employability

Truth: Seeking treatment for stress disorders or taking medical leave for exhaustion shows self-awareness and proactivity. Framing experiences with burnout as lessons in load limits can demonstrate growth to future employers.

Myth: Rest Alone Recovers Burnout

Truth: While slowing pace and resting do help remedy acute stress, burnout requires holistic rebuilding through continual boundary setting, load balancing, reframing mindsets, and healing trauma over months before fully mending. Quick fixes prove unrealistic.

Myth: Burnout Results From Weak Coping

Truth: Even the most efficient vehicles crash when operating without sufficient breaks, fuel, or maintenance. Would you blame the vehicle or the unreasonable demands put on it? Likewise, burnout is not a personal failing but rather an organizational and cultural deficit that structurally overburdens.

Myth: Burnout Only Happens Once

Truth: Recurrence proves likely when returning to identical taxing conditions without implementing lifestyle changes or securing organizational change, realigning workload capacities with humane limits. Sustainable change prevents relapses.

Myth: You Should Keep Quiet About Burnout

Truth: Breaking the silence about experiencing burnout or sharing comeback stories normalizes that this happens to even the most dedicated professionals when systems fail people. Transparency promotes cultural change.

Myth: Burnout Stigma Sticks Forever

Truth: As more leaders come forward vulnerably sharing recovery stories, understanding increases. Framing painful growth opportunities as the beginning of positive transformation dissolves limiting labels. Talk openly about the lessons learned.

Myth: Burnout Dooms Your Career

Truth: Reassessing career fit need not destroy but rather reconstruct career trajectories aligned with sustainable boundaries, fueling excellence. Reframing survival in toxic work environments as a testament to resilience and self-care commitment further showcases future assets.

Myth: Burnout Proves Rare

Truth: Unfortunately, modern epidemic levels show burnout touches almost everyone at some point, though some hide silently, fearing shame. True prevention requires shedding light on realities through open dialogue and building supportive rather than grinding company cultures.

Myth: Burnout Links Only To Work

Truth: This is a common misconception, yet states of overwhelming stress similarly stem from myriad sources like caregiving demands, grief, health challenges, and relationships. This often leaves little room to manage regular responsibilities without additional life pressures. Validate all people's pain; it is not a competition.

In summary, reconsider biases assuming burnout signals weakness rather than unsustainable systems. Reframe exhaustion from personal defect to societal opportunity, revolutionizing cultures and upholding humanity's divinity over productivity. Healing happens gradually by speaking the collective truth. What outdated assumptions require cultural change? The floor is yours...

Practical Strategies for Managing Stress and Preventing Burnout

When churning stress chronically outpaces coping capacity, even sparkling professionals risk burnout's burning embers gradually dimming former enthusiasm into slow resignation. But implementing science-backed techniques bolstering mind-body balance and contentment short-circuits harmful periods of stress before blazing out of control. Let's explore pragmatic solutions.

Tactics Alleviating Stress

In chaotic seasons, anchor equilibrium through:

- **Prioritizing restorative sleep**: Protect slumber from digital disruption. Realign natural rhythms and cognitive function.

- **Mindfulness practices**: Center awareness on the present without judgment, whether through meditative stillness, prayerful gratitude, or movement immersion like yoga, which cultivates breath and body consciousness.

- **Belly breathing**: Inhale slowly, visualizing your lungs inflating like balloons. Pause, holding your breath. Release tension in a long, audible exhale. Just 60 seconds soothes acute anxiety.

- **Reframing mindsets**: When demanding days drag optimism down, recall the bigger picture. This, too, shall pass. Write affirmations of self-compassion.

- **Time blocking**: Assign activities and set time blocks, creating structure amid chaos. Cluster similar tasks together to find flow states, then build in ample life-giving breaks to restore depleted dopamine.

- **Engaging hobbies**: Make time for simple pleasures like games with friends, and enjoying nature, crafts, music, or sports that spark joy. Laugh often; it produces mood-lifting endorphins and connection.

Pre-Emptive Burnout Prevention

When demands exceed capacity for extended periods, proactively prevent total meltdown through:

- **Noticing early warning signs**: Tune into messages from mind and body like fatigue, cynicism, or headaches hinting at support required before damage becomes chronic.

- **Scheduling self-reflection**: Block calendar time for assessing workplace wellness, judging career alignment, and clarifying core priorities centered on joy. Consider career counseling as an illuminating option.

- **Minding work-life balance**: Beyond maxing productivity, schedule space for family, self-care, passions, and purposeful rest. No crowning achievement makes up for missing what matters most.

- **Setting clear boundaries**: Communicate respectfully yet firmly regarding limitations. Say no without guilt. Disable digital notifications after hours. Clarify exactly what fuels you rather than routinely giving up your well-being by appeasing unreasonable demands.

- **Building support systems**: Identify workplace allies able to validate struggles, model healthy boundaries, or provide practical assistance in navigating tensions. Confide in loved ones offering ears and shoulders during vulnerable times rather than isolating.

- **Cultivating purpose**: Deep meaning soothes stress. When a passion projection begins to die down, realign daily efforts to personal values, making a positive impact. Or, better yet, make a job move if necessary. No paycheck warrants sanity.

- **Controlling what's controllable**: Improving any degree of agency helps get unstuck rewriting rules of engagement. Even modest influence over the schedule, delegating certain tasks, or communicating needs seeds motivation.

- **Minimizing stressors**: If particular job functions or toxic co-workers reliably ruin your day, log stress points, then strategize solutions: switch roles, set stronger boundaries, or address conflicts. Your health comes first.

- **Prioritizing holistic self-care**: Embrace lifestyle tweaks nurturing resilience like balanced eating, better sleep habits, fixed movement routines, or mindfulness practices that build the capacity to weather external variables out of our control.

- **Fostering community**: Shared struggles feel lighter. Collaborate with colleagues supporting similar values, connect consistently with the personal support network, and align with the company culture, cultivating psychological safety for all.

Untreated stress simmers into burnout over time, so implement survival strategies early and often! What pragmatic habit will you integrate first when buffering stress? Small steps prevent states of stress from becoming a way of life. Your well-being awaits diligent investments.

Part 4:

Vital Tactics for Fostering Resilience in Others and at Work

Chapter 8:
Growing Grit—Nurturing Resilience in Tomorrow's Leaders

Building resilience is so important to deal with whatever life throws at you. As the saying goes, if you fall seven times, you've got to get up eight. The adults who raise kids, like parents and teachers, really help lay the groundwork. When kids fall, these role models support them to keep going. This teaches resilience from a young age. Facing struggles is part of being human. But handling what comes your way gets easier when you learn resilience skills as a child.

Kids of all ages will face stressful times, disappointments, and failures as they grow. While tough, these moments can teach valuable lessons if guided well. Adults play a big role as kids watch how they handle challenges. If parents and teachers show kids how to bounce back from difficulties with resilience, that helps the children when their time comes to face adversity. How role models act when life gets hard passes down important life skills.

Managing emotions and being resilient go hand in hand. Kids need to learn how to identify feelings, share what's bothering them, and stay in control when upset. Caregivers play a big role by talking with children about difficult experiences and feelings. When adults show kids how to bounce back after tough times through empathy, forgiveness, gratitude, and hope, it helps those children build resistance to whatever life may bring later on. Learning to process emotions is strength training for the adversities we all face. With guidance, young people can build skills today to stay steady through whatever troubles come tomorrow.

Building resilience starts young through loving bonds and assurance of safety. Little kids don't handle big feelings well, but caring adults patiently show them. Validate what they're experiencing while also setting kind limits. Taking kids outside helps them learn skills like working with others, waiting for turns, and solving squabbles—invaluable for life. Reading together and pretend play builds thinking skills too, plus they help kids understand what's real and what's not. With guidance and imagination, even babies begin laying the foundations for handling whatever comes at them later on.

As kids grow into tweens and teens, guidance adapts too. Caregivers coach independence through problem-solving and choices with care. Parents balance new freedoms with rules fitting their age. Letting kids mess up while being there strengthens their ability to stick with problems when they get tough. Challenging negative thinking, breaking big tasks into small ones, and asking for help when needed—these habits serve kids beyond their years. Kids whose wellness matters to them through proper sleep, food, and movement develop powerful lifelong tools for strength during tough times.

Teens care deeply about friends as they face school stress, social drama, unrealistic expectations in media, and body changes. While pulling from parents, teens still need guidance and coaching through relationships, first loves, and rejections. Discovering interests through hobbies and sports builds courage for the bigger hurdles ahead. Keeping lines of communication open and trusting them makes risky times safer; teens will avoid danger and ask for help when down. With patience and understanding, parents can continue to help their children develop resilience skills that will serve them through all that life brings.

No matter their age, shielding or overprotecting children from stress can undermine resilience. Supportive caregivers empower kids to face uncertainty and adversity with the assurance that difficulty can be overcome. When kids feel reassured that stress can be survived and mistakes won't ruin them, fear doesn't win. Belief in resilience as a teacher of strength inspires getting through whatever comes. With caring help to find courage within, people naturally feel ready to take on life's ups and downs.

Kids with gumption face life prepared. Resilience guides college progress, jobs, and relationships—any bumps get navigated. These skills drive humanity's progress in amazing ways. Strong but caring, resilient people proudly carry torches forward for all. With heads high, hearts open, and hands out, each generation passes on to the next how to skillfully handle whatever comes. This legacy of strength, grace under pressure, and faith in people makes the world a little better with every resilient soul.

Shaping Resilience: The Crucial Role of Parents, Educators, and Caregivers

Being a parent is not easy. It's an endless journey full of teenage drama and filthy diapers. But all caring individuals, including parents, teachers, and coaches, have a significant impact on forming children into resilient young adults. Like a muscle, resilience requires training to overcome obstacles in life. By showing love, building trust, and letting kids spread their wings within safe bounds, adults can nurture mental toughness from toddler tantrums through turbulent teens.

The foundations of resilience start early. Babies need affection, routine, and patience to form secure attachments. Tots look to their parents for advice on how to react to failures like toppling block towers. School-aged kids watch how adults face conflict, stress, and setbacks. More than anyone, parents and caregivers shape a child's coping skills, self-esteem, and emotional tools needed to bounce back.

Guiding kids through unavoidable growing pains while allowing safe risks builds resilience. Letting a toddler feed teaches them persistence through messes. Encouraging a shy child to make a new buddy opens up social skills. Facing teen heartbreak after a breakup forces coping with the first real loss. If overprotected, kids fail to gain the skills needed to overcome adversity.

Of course, no one nails this gig perfectly. Parents have meltdowns like kids do! It's okay not to always have the right answer or fall short. Admitting mistakes shows you're human too. Laughing at your blunders relieves tension. What matters most is making up, showing forgiveness, and reassuring kids they are loved unconditionally.

Creating safe spaces for kids to open up takes patience, empathy, and listening without judgment. Provide a soft landing for hard lessons. Leading with curiosity rather than criticism encourages them to share their struggles. Establishing trust that home is a refuge makes kids more likely to avoid dangerous risks and speak up when overwhelmed.

Sometimes the simplest things build resilience the best. Making family meals a regular thing. Nightly reading before bedtime. Sunday hikes to unplug. Fixing up old cars together. Cooking or building side-by-side nets quality time without distractions. Shared traditions reinforce reliability kids can count on as they grow up.

When adults model self-care, kids intuitively follow. Finding work-life balance, getting enough sleep, making exercise fun, and fueling up on nutritious foods all provide the blueprint for kids to follow. Unwinding through hobbies also sets examples. Ignoring comparisons on social media teaches positive body image too. Self-care matters—trying to pour from an empty cup? You won't get very far.

Kids aren't so different from adults. Who doesn't want to belong, feel capable of pursuing their passions, and have a voice in decisions? Providing chances to join groups like sports teams or school clubs can build self-esteem. Community service nurtures purpose and citizenship. Part-time jobs teach responsibility while earning independence.

As kids grow, adults must adapt support to fit changing needs. Keep nurturing resilience over the long haul. That whiny baby will quickly mature into a competent, compassionate leader who can manage any challenge. Though no one said it would be simple, this profession might be the most fulfilling one available.

Common Challenges

Since most people don't even know what resilience is, raising resilient children may be challenging. In essence, it's the capacity to overcome adversity and disappointment. Kids aren't born with it naturally; it's shaped over time with help from caring adults. As a result, parents, teachers, and coaches play a huge role. But it isn't easy guiding kids through growing pains to cope well when life gets messy.

First, understanding resilience helps adults nurture it better. Take the time to realize kids need support facing fears, adapting to change, and overcoming obstacles bit by bit. Know that some anxiety is normal. She struggles as a growth opportunity. Model optimistic thinking. Reach out when you need a hand too.

Providing secure environments gives kids roots to spread their wings. Make your home a refuge to unwind, laugh, and chat over meals. Build trust with your kids so they open up and avoid dangerous risks. Give them chances to make choices so they learn from outcomes. Set kind, firm limits so they don't crumble under too much freedom too soon. Move at their pace.

Promoting open communication takes time and empathy, without judgment. Lead with curiosity instead of criticism. Let kids express all their feelings freely. Admit when you mess up too. Listen without immediately providing quick fixes to build insight. See issues from their angle without dismissing their views. Reassure them and offer your support, no matter what.

Teaching kids to regulate emotions well is hard but worth it. From toddler tantrums to teen drama, labeling complex feelings helps with processing. Guiding intense anger into healthy outlets prevents harm. Model good emotion regulation and apologize after the dust settles. Don't shame crybabies but comfort them. Praise every small step and manage frustrations well.

Nothing replaces nurturing human connections. Schedule dedicated time without digital distractions. Snuggling small kids into bed soothes pains and worries. Share in their proud moments and dreams for the future. Laugh off embarrassing blunders to relieve tension. Build traditions to reinforce reliability.

Modeling adult resilience shows kids how it's done. Voice positive self-talk and face your struggles. Ask peers for help when work problems pile up. Start new hobbies to flex creativity. Prepare healthy snacks to manage stress. Plugging into spiritual practices keeps perspective.

In hard times, instilling optimistic thinking lifts spirits. When plans crumble, brainstorm solutions together. After failures, emphasize lessons learned. Count the little blessings in the gloom. Support their dreams through unsure futures. When kids see you keep hopeful despite troubles, it inspires their outlook tremendously.

The lack of supportive adults in a kid's life can majorly disrupt emotional growth. Single parents stretched thin to make ends meet and can't provide the quality time needed. Friends couch surfing at unstable homes disrupts the basis for resilience. Teachers bogged with large classes can miss signs of bullying. Overstressed caregivers can snap to harsh reactions that shame tender spirits.

Guiding kids patiently to solve their problems equips them with life skills. Instead of fixing dilemmas for them, ask, "What ideas might improve this situation?" Strategizing options together builds confidence. Reflecting on choices that escalated versus resolving conflicts nurtures wisdom for next time.

Many kids today lack chances to play freely, exploring their imagination and social abilities. Tightly structured days shuffle them from school to extracurriculars with little free time to just chill. Excess screen time overstimulates minds, limiting in-person interaction. Overprotecting kids from minor risks hinders building common sense. Allowing beginner independence provides small wins vital for growth.

No parent has this gig nailed 100%, but doing your best is enough. Shower kids with compassion. Foster intrinsically motivating hobbies. Limit compare and despair messages from the media. Model self-care, which is indispensable for pouring from a full cup. Laugh on days when it all goes wrong. Make amends after blowing a fuse too fast. Replay often: Kids spell love by T-I-M-E—keep making deposits into emotional banks!

Solutions

Did you know 9.4% of kids between the ages of 3 and 17 were diagnosed with anxiety between 2016 and 2019 (Centers for Disease Control and Prevention, 2019)? 25.1% of children between the ages of 13 and 18 are estimated to have an anxiety condition (Wang et al., 2017).

Raising kids to bounce back from life's bumps isn't easy, but you don't have to figure it out alone. With so many demands, it's normal to get overwhelmed. When patience runs thin, take a timeout to regroup. Lean on other parents to swap ideas or just vent. And have compassion for yourself when parental guilt creeps in!

Learning about resilience gives insight into kids' brain development. Their emotions and logic skills aren't mature yet. Read up on age-appropriate ways to boost adaptive coping. Check if schools offer classes helping kids handle anxiety, anger, or grief. Knowledge is power!

Little daily actions create a secure environment where kids open up. Greet them first thing with a hug. Ask engaging questions at dinnertime. Limit electronics before bedtime to chat instead. Schedule weekly dates to connect one-on-one without distraction. Post inspiring quotes and family photos displaying unconditional love.

Better communication starts with listening and observing before reacting. Allow all feelings to be expressed without judgment. Lead with empathy and validation before giving advice. Admit when you flub up, that models humility. Discuss managing disagreements respectfully. Send encouraging notes in lunchboxes to reinforce support.

Equipping kids with healthy coping tools pays off in the long term. Teach calming practices like deep belly breathing, visualization, mindfulness, or yoga. Play soothing music to relax before bed. Model positive self-talk when you feel disappointed. Vocalize your gratitude during tough times. Laugh together and blow off steam through silliness.

Nothing replaces one-on-one nurturing care from trusted adults. Schedule individual-focused activities like crafting, baking, or yardwork together. Share proud moments that shape identity. Regularly verbalize your unconditional love and belief in them. Institute weekly check-ins to gauge emotional tanks without pressure.

Kids watch your resilience in the face of setbacks. Voice the self-talk and problem-solving that happen in your head when facing worries. Ask peers for support in managing work stress. Take quiet breaks to regroup when overwhelmed before reacting. Show accountability and how to make amends after conflicts. Discuss what resilience or perseverance means through examples kids relate to.

If you see a child struggling without adequate adult support at home or school, reach out. Coach overwhelmed parents on self-care and building resilience. Help teachers spot and assist vulnerable students slipping through the cracks. Ask how you can volunteer if a family you know is in crisis through job loss, health issues, or other hardship.

Instead of rescuing kids from issues, guide them to tackle manageable challenges. Break big problems into step-by-step plans. Reinforce trying new strategies if they get stuck. Ask empowering questions like, "What part can you handle even if you mess up?" Base confidence on effort rather than perfect outcomes. Praise every small win!

Make space for regular playtime where kids direct imaginative activities while you participate. Welcome their ideas and follow their lead. Avoid criticizing performance. Instead, enjoy laughter, adventure, and relationship building. Foster personal motivation through their unique interests without pushing for structured outcomes.

There is no need to pressure yourself to strive for "perfect parent" status. Sprinkle love and nurturing care into your days however you can. Laugh and make goofy memories at dance parties. Share your favorite book series. Train pets with fun new tricks. Display art projects with pride. Post-glow-in-the-dark stars for bedroom dreaming.

Understanding Resilience in Different Age Groups

Resilience helps kids bounce back from life's curveballs and setbacks. But it looks pretty different as young ones grow from precious preschoolers to moody middle schoolers and beyond. Understanding what resilience building blocks suit each age sets realistic expectations for ourselves and our kids.

In early childhood, (from toddlerhood to age eight) little ones mainly need oodles of comfort and support. Their brains grow rapidly, yet they lack logic and emotional control. Like sponges, they soak up lessons on reacting appropriately to challenges by watching caregivers closely.

Say your tiny tots topple block towers in frustration. Rather than shame their meltdowns, offer hugs and firmly say why hitting is unkind. Recognize that words fail when emotions run high! Set limits; give space to cry or scream into pillows. Then redirect play to teach flexibility through pretend scenarios.

Around preschool, kids start learning simple coping techniques but forget them quickly when upset. Remind them to take deep breaths or count to five when anger bubbles. The role model apologizes to dollies when they react with tantrums too. Build memory through repetition and patience as their brains develop.

In this stage, resilience sprouts from secure attachments at home and with teachers. Eat meals together and makeup games about overcoming adversity. Snuggle worries away at bedtime, then review in daylight optimism. A balance between giving affection and respecting independent play is also needed.

Around the age six, the school introduces fresh stressors like competition, peer drama, and academic pressure. Navigate disappointment over poor grades with encouragement to keep trying new strategies. Spot signs of bullying early and alert staff to promote safe classrooms for all.

In middle childhood, spanning ages 9 to 12, kids better understand resilience concepts but still look to adults for support when facing intensified hardship. Competition in academics and sports can eat away at self-confidence without effort to redirect focus on self-improvement rather than besting peers. Tweens may hide embarrassing challenges like acne teasing or exclusion from friend groups, so create safe spaces to share upsets. Where age is appropriate, guide the tween through advocacy for their own needs to build decision-making skills. Share stories about overcoming your adversity and respect how things feel much larger through their lens. Affirm that there's no right way to show resilience; meeting kids where they are with love matters most.

As kids enter adolescence, beginning around age 13, peer approval feels essential to identity. Allow teens to take safe risks to explore independence within protective boundaries. Making small decisions like budgeting allowance, arranging schedules, or redecorating bedrooms promotes capable life skills, even when they flub. Boost resilience by allowing failure and then providing support to process disappointment through journaling, art, or heart-to-heart conversations. Caregiver modeling self-care techniques like exercise, nutrition, and unplugged downtime influences teen behavior more than nagging ever could.

While teens pull away, seeking privacy, remain present and approachable. Neutrally suggest thinking through consequences when you spot high-risk behaviors. Ask teens' opinions on family issues to reinforce your faith in their growing wisdom. Support identity development through praise, displaying creative work, or recalling proud moments. Though eye rolls abound, your unconditional love and guidance are still priceless lifelines, even if unacknowledged.

No matter a child's age, resilience relies on caregiving bonds established over the years through affection, communication, and support. Have patience with little ones as their abilities slowly improve to express and manage emotions. Respect expanding independence in adolescents while keeping your door open when they need reassurance only a caring adult can provide. Foster resilience across all stages through empowering love.

Growing Strong: Strategies for Boosting Resilience in Youth

Growing kids' resilience requires suiting their changing needs, from precious preschoolers to tempestuous teens. Tailoring support by age equips them to get back up when life knocks them down. These key strategies used by counselors and educators build mental muscle throughout childhood.

For tiny tots from three to eight years old, make connections through one-on-one play, reading together, and chatting over meals. Get on their level, literally, to role model reacting appropriately when frustrated. Label and validate big feelings to increase emotional awareness. Redirect overflowing excitement or anger into healthy outlets like Play-Doh pounding or goofing around with water.

Encourage toddlers to help shoulder simple chores matching their abilities to boost their self-confidence. Set up stepstools to reach sinks for hand washing or toy bins for clean-up. Recognize effort over perfection with high fives. Being helpful and reliable gives young kids purpose.

Maintaining consistent naptime, mealtime, and bedtime routines provides comfort. Display visual schedule reminders. Ease transitions by counting down to the next activity. Consistency and predictability lower distress when unfamiliar or stressful situations arise.

Support free emotional expression without judgment. Never shame cries, tantrums, or nightmares, but set limits on aggression. Teach calming techniques like belly breathing and coloring while music plays softly. Create cozy spaces for meltdowns with stuffed animal friends on hand to soothe. Validating feelings helps toddlers own and eventually regulate big reactions.

Model resilience when you mess up or face daily stressors. Voice positive self-talk out loud: "That was so frustrating! It's ok; I can try again." Verbalize your process openly. Explain how you regain optimism in tough times. Kids mimic coping strategies they repeatedly observe, just like speech patterns.

Lastly, promote child-led play, allowing imagination and social skills to flourish freely. Set dress-ups, blocks, and craft supplies ready for exploration rather than overly programming each minute. Facilitate sharing, and resolve conflicts calmly. Fostering unstructured play now encourages later innovation, executive function, and adaptability.

In middle childhood, from ages 9–12, peer relationships gain importance alongside school achievement. Develop kids' social abilities by modeling how to join groups, take turns, and compromise. Role play: starting conversations, responding to exclusion, and destructive gossip or bullying. Build confidence through community service projects.

Combat rising performance pressure and comparisons by reframing your thoughts. When kids label themselves failures after setbacks, reframe gently, "That test felt impossible, but remember those times you kept practicing something tough until you got it!" Remind yourself that brains keep developing, so new strategies work over time.

Around 4th–6th grade, independence surges but still needs guidance. Allow goal-setting, then periodic check-ins on progress. Permit choices like packing their lunch or managing homework time. Stand back, offering support only when truly stuck. Small wins foster intrinsic motivation.

Apply emerging logic skills to tackle problems collaboratively. On conflicts with peers, ask, "What are some ways we could have shared the toy more fairly?" Strategize solutions to anxiety before music recitals or tests. Break overwhelming tasks into steps to gain traction.

Support physical activity through games, family bike rides, or participating in sports teams to reduce worries. Exercise naturally improves mood and the ability to focus. Set healthy habits through meal prep together. Discuss balancing digital fun with unplugged hobbies to recharge.

In adolescence (ages 13–19), peer belonging critically impacts self-esteem. Encourage open communication to facilitate support. Normalize seeking counseling for mental health needs without stigma. Discuss resolving relational conflicts directly rather than venting online. Set reasonable restrictions on youth social media use.

Teach healthy coping mechanisms to help big emotions not overwhelm. Journaling, creative arts, and physical outlets let teens process internal stress. Mindfulness apps ease anxiety. Volunteer work promotes meaning and community when loneliness looms. Assure them that counselors can aid serious crises confidentially.

Through later teens, guide goal-setting for training, college, and jobs. Map plans out, adjusting for strengths, challenges, and economic realities. Break intimidating steps into a timeline, like saving for car insurance, to gain freedom. Review budgets, balancing wants, and fiscal wisdom. Praise diligent effort toward realistic ambitions.

Promote self-care as indispensable, not selfish or vain. Model limiting compare and despair messages from media and peers. Discuss managing unhealthy parties and substance pressures. Recommend online wellness advice from teens' trusted celebrities. Validate needed autonomy within the protective concern, not control.

It helps teens to gain a sense of purpose and contribution. Explore career mentoring that matches their passion. Cheer community chorus performances. Visit colleges that specialize in related fields to inspire big dreams. Recognize causes they care about and encourage problem-solving ideas to support making a difference at any age.

The Power of Fostering Healthy Physical Coping

When kids get overwhelmed by big feelings, blowing off steam physically can work wonders. Instead of bottling frustrations that might erupt in tantrums or tuning out through constant electronics, show them to let the energy flow in healthy ways. Teaching simple practices early helps emotional regulation as they grow.

Young kids, especially, have limitless energy and limited self-control. Getting the wiggles out constructively prevents acting out and reduces anxiety. Physical outlets improve mood through brain chemicals and a sense of capability and mastery skills. Connecting movement to emotions makes the lesson stick better, too.

Turn tense times into a silly "squeeze-relax" game. Have kids scrunch up their faces, hunch their shoulders to their ears, and clench their fists tightly for five seconds. Then abruptly shout "Relax!" prompting them to release all tension and flop limp. Laughing along helps; do multiple rounds until the room lightens up.

For school-aged kids overwhelmed by stimuli and thoughts, lead a "5-4-3-2-1 grounding exercise. Look around, naming five things you see, four things you feel, three things you hear, two things that smell, and one that tastes good, like peppermint. It redirects rushing thoughts to calmer present-moment awareness.

In moments of conflict or defiance, inject fun through playful challenges. Call out dance moves like "Tiptoe left, spin right, jump up high!" Foster listening skills by having them lead you through the next round of actions. For snappy teens, make a hand-squeezing contest, then arm wrestle across the table to reset moods with laughter.

Developing daily habits using physical outlets allows for safe emotional release. Make encouraging fitness fun rather than forcing exercise that feels like punishment. Allow choices based on changing interests to stick with motivation.

Turn on upbeat music for morning jump rope contests. Assign point values for skips, crisscrosses, and alternated foot patterns. Tally scores through the week, building endurance. Form hula-hoop relay race teams in the yard for giggles.

Shoot hoops together to see who can score the most creative baskets—bonus points for backward over the head! Turn chores like unloading groceries or raking leaves into team weightlifting challenges. Walk the dog around new neighborhood blocks, discovering adventure.

Set up obstacle courses indoors or outdoors, challenging their speed, reactions, and problem-solving. Crawl under tables, hop sideways over sticks, and balance along curb edges. Time attempts pacing yourself, then sprint again pursuing personal bests. Building body awareness and capability creates confidence to handle tougher life obstacles ahead too.

Allow teens outlets like jogging, dance classes, or skateboarding groups for social bonding beyond school. Encourage finding recreational community teams or outdoor adventure trips that match individual strengths for connection. Guiding as a mentor, not a critic, is key; highlighting growth, not gaps in personal motivation.

For younger kids, set up stations for bouncing basketballs, blowing bubbles, and pinwheels for gross motor (physical) fun and development. Work multiple senses, helping emotional regulation. Have mini trampoline contests to see who pops bubbles with the coolest tricks. Let imagination soar freely, chasing bubbles far and wide!

Any good mood-boosting tactic worth learning gets practiced when emotions run high until it becomes a natural habit. Role model healthy movement yourself to relieve stress—maybe by just admitting you have the wiggles today and doing a silly wiggle dance together. Releasing mental and physical tension frees up energy to handle situations better going forward.

The Power of Fostering Healthy Emotional Coping

Kids absorb so much through their environments—for better and worse. While we can't shield them from pain, we can equip them with healthy responses. When big feelings seem too much, emotional tools help you regroup. Teaching coping strategies early on builds lifelong resilience.

The power of positivity can't be overstated. Despite hardship, maintaining a hopeful vision fuels perseverance. Guide kids in rehearsing optimistic self-talk to reframe setbacks as growth opportunities. Affirm, "I know you can handle this!" to cultivate grit during inevitable failures. Your reassuring voice echoes in their minds in future trials.

Simple breathing exercises tap into the body's built-in stress relief system. Have anxious kids inhale slowly through the nose for five counts. Purse your lips tightly while forcefully exhaling six counts. Repeat a few cycles until the shoulders relax. The extra exhale time activates the calming parasympathetic nervous system.

For variety, instruct kids to trace rainbow arcs through the air, deliberately inhaling ascending red to violet, then exhaling descending violet to red. Vivid visualization combined with movement focuses attention away from worries. Or have them imagine smelling delicious pizza cooking—deep inhalations via the nose and long blows out of the mouth. Make it a game until smiles return.

Unleashing feelings through the creative arts fosters self-awareness and emotional intelligence. Keep journals handy for recording thoughts and dreams. Doodle worries away, scribbling freely; no art skill is required! Craft individual worry stones that kids rub when anxious. Customize a "calm down" jar with glitter swirls settling as music plays softly.

Turn on your favorite tunes and dance, drum, or sing out loud—maybe with funny improvised lyrics about problems. Show that it's okay to be silly and imperfect. Creating beauty out of struggles builds resilience. Display masterpieces prominently to reinforce your capability to face challenges ahead.

Words hold power, for good and bad. After scoldings, notice if negative self-talk replays unnecessarily harshly in kids' minds. To counter, teach positive affirmations created collectively. Write "I am strong," "Challenges make me grow," or "My family loves me no matter what" on cards placed in backpacks and lunch boxes for quick reminders!

Model healthy emotional responses when facing your upsets. Label anger, sadness, or disappointment when they strike rather than hiding stress. Take a walk around the block to process important conversations. Play soft piano music to self-soothe through grief. Verbalize thinking through upsetting conflicts out loud. Kids emulate strategies we demonstrate far more than just telling them about it.

No one handles hard times gracefully every time. When emotions erupt, don't shame kids. Stop hurtful actions firmly yet gently. Offer empathy for overwhelming feelings after all settles. Analyze together: What heated the situation? How can we communicate better next time? Support kids owning and resolving regrets through restorative conversation, amends, or acts of service.

Learning occurs best when emotions aren't running high. Revisit upsetting experiences once calm, analyzing what triggered reactions. Discuss how peers might perceive overlapping perspectives. Brainstorm more positive responses if situations repeat themselves. Write thank-you notes to teachers, coaches, and friends after conflicts. Moving forward with intention prevents hanging onto resentment.

Just like reading or math skills, coping techniques improve with devoted practice when the stakes feel low. Role-play responding to mistakes or bullying. Rehearse managing worries through journaling, music, and breathing. Develop personalized strategies that resonate most with each child's unique personality. Over time, self-regulation becomes an effortless habit to draw upon when adversity strikes in the years ahead.

Chapter 9:
Thriving Amid Turbulence—Building Resilience in the Workplace

The winds of change blow fiercely in the modern workplace. Advancing technology and automation will transform job roles overnight. Economic booms and busts shake industries without warning. The Great Resignation highlights how priorities have shifted toward purpose and flexibility in exchange for loyalty. Amid such uncertainty and change, the ability to adapt and bounce back from disruptions determines professional success and satisfaction now more than ever before.

Resilience provides an invisible backbone when outside circumstances feel out of our control. Viewing change as an opportunity builds optimism and fuels progress. Managing the stress of ambiguity and conflict prevents burnout. Achieving greater work-life balance and self-care sustains energy for the long haul. While some naturally handle turbulence better than others, resilience can be intentionally nurtured.

Progress depends on responding wisely when plans hit snags. Proactively preparing contingency plans when launching initiatives ensures you are both focused and flexible. Detaching ego from outcomes reminds us that worth is not defined by each win or loss on the journey. Reframing moments of crisis into windows for innovation and growth is an empowering perspective.

Of course, even dedicated professionals have natural physical and emotional limits over time. Without proper rest, nutrition, and renewal, even the most passionate employee will crumble. The built-up impact of stress magnifies when our fuel storage runs empty. Thus, companies promoting wellness practices through staff mental health days, workplace counseling, and developmental workshops enjoy higher retention and efficiency.

Creating work cultures where employees encourage one another through challenges produces richer human connections. People who feel valued and equipped with leadership skills carry these strengths into community roles outside of office walls. Investing in each person's growth around resilience and ethics pays exponential dividends across society for generations to come.

Now more than ever before, the ability to adapt, learn continuously, and collaborate with empathy are non-negotiable leadership skills as technology and markets accelerate faster than schools can keep pace. Yet human nature instinctively resists change, filters perspectives through personal bias, and fails to recharge. With aspiration, discipline, and compassion, a thriving workplace is possible even amid turbulence.

Workplace Resilience: A Key to Professional Triumph

Navigating work life isn't easy these days. Changes blow in fiercely as digital disruption transforms job skills overnight. Hustling harder to stand out is draining. Cutthroat competition erodes loyalty between peers. Maintaining balance feels just out of reach. How do people not just survive but thrive amid nonstop crazy workplace turbulence? That's where developing resilience saves our sanity—and careers.

Resilience is adapting well when situations get rocky. Instead of crumbling, you flex. Challenges feel manageable, not paralyzing because you expect to change and know you can handle it. Resilient people stay solution-focused and ask for help to work smarter. They press forward with optimism, believing growth opportunities bloom even in storms.

Toughness matters a ton when change hits constantly across industries. Tech disrupts how we work; automation alters tasks. Colleagues switch companies, chasing better perks. Budget cuts or mergers shake departments overnight. Rapid restructuring means nonstop uncertainty and stress for all.

Amid the chaos, resilience provides professional superpowers from within. Laughing at setbacks prevents cynicism. Standing tall through unfair criticism builds confidence to take calculated risks that pay off down the road. Bouncing back from burnout lets you encourage exhausted teammates in time.

Simply put, resilience enhances overall well-being—mental, physical, and emotional health. You cope better when plans crumble because your worth isn't defined just by work success. Focusing on what's controllable and letting go of what's not brings freedom from anxiety. Deeper self-knowledge helps set boundaries, preventing exhaustion. You realize it quicker when it's time to walk away from toxic situations that damage your peace of mind. Protecting inner joy lets you keep others from taking it away from you.

Resilience boosts adaptability, helping change feel exciting and not threatening. Failures become feedback to tweak strategies. You brainstorm creative workarounds when obstacles loom rather than freeze. Flexibility lets you rebound quickly from flesh wounds. Being always teachable makes you tougher rather than fragile—actually, you gain strength through dealing with tough situations. This finesse will only become more career-critical as technological speed accelerates.

When tensions build up between colleagues or sales quarter goals prove difficult to reach, resilient professionals stay solution-focused. Laser vision zooms in on the most important action steps. Team harmony is restored through acknowledging all perspectives. Road mapping multiple scenarios proactively prepares us. Peace spreads through a non-anxious presence, even when facing worries.

Over the long haul, resilient teams simply produce greater results—plain and simple. Energy gets channeled into opportunity zones, not dragged down by pessimists. People pull together, aligning strengths for multiplied impact. Passion fuels late nights when sudden changes require all hands on deck. Customer retention skyrockets thanks to responsive service surpassing expectations.

Strong connections strengthen teams when circumstances threaten unity. Celebrating tiny wins together sparks intrinsic motivation that outperforms cash incentives alone. Having each other's backs through sickness, new parenthood, or family loss builds loyalty beyond payroll. Shared respect remains rock steady, whether stock options dive or rise. Constructive conflict fuels creativity and success without tearing at the fabric of relationships. Resilience glues relationships where rewards and roles flex continually.

For leaders aspiring for growth, resilience builds key emotional intelligence skills that set them apart. Communicating with compassion, not condescension is the difference between poor leaders and true visionaries. Admitting knowledge gaps and seeking solutions humbly creates trust and respect. Empathizing with staff struggles while providing unconditional support nurtures loyalty, and ensures that they will do the same for you.

Mentally preparing for nonstop change ultimately breeds confidence by chasing bold career moves rather than clinging to security blankets. Transferable resilience skills bridge the transition between passions—from teacher to real estate investor or engineer to startup founder. Becoming adaptable lets you embrace the adventure of reinvention without the stabilizers others depend on to feel safe.

Bottom line: resilience empowers us to expect turbulence yet believe in better days ahead. Mental adaptability helps weather workplace storms without losing hope or heart in the process. Invest in building resilience within yourself and your teams for fruitful seasons destined to bloom after floods eventually dry up.

Unmasking Common Challenges and Stressors

Some work stress is just part of life: deadlines loom, competitors bite at our heels, and changes demand learning new software or safety protocols. However, employers allowing excessive strains to damage employee health costs everyone and it only builds up over time. Ignoring toxic stressors eats away at our engagement, caps creativity that strengthens revenue, and gives star players a reason to jump ship fast. As much as individuals must build resilience by adapting to daily strains, organizational leadership shares responsibility for fostering environments where people energize each other and do not drain scarce reserves bone dry. The most successful work cultures promote holistic human health, realizing that sustainable results depend as much on safe psychological spaces as ergonomic desk setups and snack bars.

Let's call out commonly destructive stress culprits stealing vibrant morale day by day. Unrealistic deadlines that demand regular overtime sap mental clarity, physical stamina, and emotional mood-boosting chemicals like serotonin. Feelings of never achieving enough erupt even in able professionals, who self-identify as failures despite their real contributions. Allowing sufficient scheduling, reasonable goal expectations, and celebrating small milestones protects against prolonged exhaustion that turns high performers toward apathy and cynicism over time.

Stress multiplies when policies change at a whim without explanation or input, and those changes disrupt. Firings mean survivors must absorb more roles for no increased compensation, which strains already low energy banks past their capacity. Mergers disrupting established team rhythms and norms inject anxiety that lingers distractingly. Even positive expansions like acquiring trendy new equipment stretch workers to learn updated programs fast amid already-packed workloads. Leadership owes transparent communication around changing expectations before dropping news that sabotages stability vital for focus.

When job security wavers precariously, so does the loyal worker's commitment to advance company visions versus protecting their livelihoods first. Fearful workers reasonably keep ideas to themselves to shine individually, especially if peer collaboration might strengthen a competitor's resume. Why invest in team building when camaraderie could be cut off suddenly by layoffs? Reasonable reassurances around restructuring intentions restore an authentic community where everyone protects each other and rises together.

Overburdened workloads and crushing work-life balance long-term builds hidden resentment waiting to surface when stress bubbles over. People struggling in isolation blame circumstances instead of seeking creative alternatives. Does shifting meetings to start later accommodate commuting parents? Could budgets allow freelance support during peak demand periods? Even small accommodations that relieve excessive demands breed loyalty and passionate ownership for company success.

When colleagues compete aggressively, protecting individual advancement, environments build anxiety rather than trust to build healthy connections. Whether through misunderstandings, selfish motivations, or outright sabotage, difficult co-workers drain precious energy. Seeking root issues through open dialogue or addressing tensions through neutral conversation redirects focus on shared goals, not personalized differences that divide.

Micromanagers squashing the independence required for innovative solutions communicates distrust more than support to overwhelmed workers. The best coaches empower appropriate independence guided by a common vision; overcontrolling supervision backfires by limiting potential. Leaders clarifying a bigger purpose and then allowing flexible freedom to direct customized tactics allow game-changing ideas to grow.

Boredom is as energy-depleting over time as a chaotic frenzy for quick learners who thrive on novelty and creative challenges. Lackluster tasks repeated in monotony kill the passion for making a positive impact that attracted top talent in the first place. Roles built too heavily on routine slowly disenchant high achievers whose strengths shine in creating better systems, not just maintaining mediocrity. Inviting suggestions and restructuring workflow prevents staleness from eating away at peak contributors' self-actualization and performance over time.

Unclear instructions waste critical time by obsessively double-checking the next steps, fearing corrections later. Whether hurriedly communicated or lacking structured processes, unclear objectives create anxiety when delivered. Consistent processes with well-communicated protocols ensure high quality and efficiency. Be sure handbooks and training match workflows for easy cooperation. Updated policies and anticipating audience questions ahead of time erase confusion before it spirals.

Perhaps against one's expectations, some dread emerges from excessively high-performance expectations without margins that are ever quite sufficient. Parental pressure to achieve excellence carries over unconsciously. Perfectionists driving at a relentless pace can spark inspiration yet risk burnout without proper recovery. Internalizing self-worth as linked to productivity ignores human limitations requiring rest. Manage unrealistic standards with compassion, balancing self-care, and ambitious targets to sustain positive results lifelong.

Where leadership allows unhealthy attitudes around interaction, performance evaluation, work-life balance, or diversity, the best talent seeks healthier ecosystems elsewhere. Workers feel disrespected or neglected, delivering the minimal effort required without ever having their hearts in it. On the flip side, organizations prioritizing people as multidimensional individuals with care and calling far beyond their cubicles alone earn strong loyalty in return. The choice is clear: nourish human souls or watch dreams wither!

The Impact of Workplace Stressors

Workplace stress is inevitable—we aren't robots after all. But excessive, unrelenting pressures eat away at even the toughest spirits, kept too long on adrenaline's razor edge. As health spirals, so do engagement and performance, which companies depend on. Stopping neglect before it necessitates serious intervention both prevents reduceable disease burdens and protects bottom lines threatened by lowered output or turnover fleeing toxic settings.

Unmanaged tensions manifest through physical symptoms first, raising alarms that something mentally isn't right. Sleep disrupted by racing thoughts or midnights spent obsessing over worries revs up stress hormones, leaving immune systems vulnerable. Caffeine and sugar can act as bandages, but they only worsen the vicious cycles. Sports injuries and sickness sideline previously consistent gym goers, who suddenly inactive and dissatisfied.

Migraines from eyestrain squinting at computers too long turn weekend downtime into painful rest periods rather than restorative ones. Headaches pulse incessantly while we massage tender necks knotted with worry. Jaw soreness accompanies clenched teeth as we obsess over difficult interactions and conversations we need to have.

Digestive troubles mean that easy foods become triggers for bloating, acid reflux, and irritable bowels. Ulcers develop over months when churning acid eats away at the intestinal lining, struggling to process inflammation caused by stress. Struggling without relief eats away at confidence and competence, spiraling downward.

Unmanaged stress notoriously manifests through cardiovascular impacts such as raised blood pressure, irregular heart rhythms, and aggravated cholesterol levels. Early indicators like shortness of breath, heart palpitations, or dizzy spells warn that vascular systems are clogged under thickening plaque, and disrupted by cortisol's blood vessel constriction. What begins as occasional discomfort can lead to full-blown heart attacks or strokes through cumulative damage over the years.

Alongside obvious physical cues, hiding away emotional stress and worries only sabotages work relationships and performance. This can be subtle but equally dangerously long-term. Anxiety and feelings of being overwhelmed narrowly focus on putting out immediate fires rather than a strategic vision for the future. Knee-jerk reactions keep us scared and unaligned with the organizational values we once upheld. Sensitive situations trigger overreacting outbursts or retreats into withdrawn isolation.

Uncharacteristic mood swings, irrational irritability, and emotional struggles alienate colleagues who previously enjoyed our company. Project planning falls hostage to unreliability from shortened fuses and a lack of follow-through. Cynicism and feelings of futility poison previously upbeat attitudes until negativity feels normal.

Prolonged uncertainty gives way to clinical depression, sapping energy, and clouding futures once brightly hopeful. Passion fizzles through perpetual fatigue, struggling just to finish basic tasks, much less creative collaboration. Isolation increases the absence of fun friendships that fueled community before. Leaders, overwhelmed by themselves, run on empty legs with nothing left to inspire teams.

Careers depend equally on political capital through networking and trust as tangible skills. But strained relationships have heavy costs personally and professionally when stress exceeds healthy thresholds. Kind leaders grow cold, speaking through restrained hostility, and not understanding empathy. Star performers quietly disengage, their productivity fading first before ultimately quitting, demoralized.

Invisible exhaustion caps the strategic thinking required to solve complex challenges. Poor judgment due to stress risks client dissatisfaction through overlooked details once easily managed. Disorganization weakens efficiency by having us always scrambling. Poor memory means important messages slip through the cracks, unanswered amid overflowing inboxes.

Stress fills cups already at maximum capacity until health suffers through built-up strain. Physiological symptoms nudge us towards attempting restorative self-care, but demands outpace those resources. Still, without systemic change that reinforces boundaries, individuals hardly stand a chance.

The good news is that through resetting cultural norms and priorities at an organizational level, daily stresses can be balanced, preventing this landslide into burnout. But first, companies must acknowledge excessive workplace strain as a preventable indicator of unsustainability, not an isolated weakness of individuals. Healing starts with leaders empowering authenticity about struggles, and then demonstrating holistic support through life's inevitable ups and downs.

The alternative path continues to demoralize talented teams, who are resigning to find more life-giving environments. Unique skill sets honed through years of work cannot simply be replaced overnight through quick turnover. Phrases like "People quit managers, not jobs" reveal that misplaced accountability continues to drive away human capital, the most valuable long-run corporate asset.

Prioritizing sustainable pacing over rapid expansion protects infrastructure beyond quarterly fluctuations. Honoring an employee's full and many-layered lives outside office walls leverages passion and creativity unlocked when given proper room and time to refuel. Companies insisting workers leave health and souls at the entry gates wonder why their once innovative ideas and soaring stock prices stop over time.

Renewed energy surges by rehumanizing workplaces one conversation at a time. Start listening today before blood pressure medications and shrinking patent pipelines sound the loudest alarms. Prevention sustains advantages, growing over time when commitment also builds up long-term.

They say stress kills slowly in the darkness before you ever spot it creeping up. But glaring red flags wave right under our noses if we know what to look for. Subtle changes in thinking, emotions, behaviors, and relationships signal burnout brewing beneath the surface. Intervening early and adjusting unreasonable workloads prevents crises later after health deteriorates. Promoting mental wellness enhances lives now and safeguards future growth, benefiting all in the long term.

Intellectual signals first emerge subtly through losing concentration that once was laser-focused on deliverables, not distractions. Scattered thoughts pass through rapidly without properly finding insights from them. Forgetfulness multiplies until constant uncertainty undermines the confidence to lead boldly. Details fall through the cracks unnoticed, prompting embarrassing corrections and wasting precious time.

Procrastination skyrockets as mundane tasks feel meaningless without a clarified purpose. Passions that attract top talent drift tiredly through an uninspiring routine. Ambitious ideas left unpursued slowly die amid the crushing bureaucracies. Phones buzz repeatedly, unanswered when quotas replace action.

Overwhelming short circuits and logical reasoning are desperately needed to navigate complex dilemmas. Flustered minds default to reactionary judgments, despite years of experience and schooling. Disorganization prevents smoothly implementing initiatives that were once effortlessly managed. Impulsive decisions lack proper calculation, ones that would be evident if properly rested. Delays and costs to redo poor work multiply until inefficiencies demand serious evaluation.

Unresolved knots eventually damage relationships that were once easily collaborative. Miscommunications create resentment that builds up without open dialogue. Blaming replaces seeking shared responsibility. Defensive postures prevent solutions, and losing sight of mutual goals. Isolation increases when the camaraderie that once sparked ingenuity and accountability is gone.

Overstressed individuals often cope by dangerously hiding symptoms temporarily through unhealthy means. Reliant alcohol use soars, numbing cares that haunt endlessly. Midday drinks sneak alcohol tolerance higher until real addiction takes hold. Professionalism suffers when intoxication impairs interactions and mood stability.

Libidos flatline through stress, even though the intimate connections offer safe harbors amid storms. Partners ache from not observing laughter, and affection slowly dies through emotional absence rather than presence. Exhaustion replaces exhilaration, robbing precious moments shared by unwinding together. Evenings spent zoning out on devices erase opportunities for reconnecting and releasing daily tension.

Stoic leaders explode unexpectedly when stretched beyond healthy limits over the years, repressing their reactions. Rage surfaces sharply without restraint, shocking colleagues unfamiliar with such furious outbursts over minor things. Harsh overcorrections require extensive repairs to reestablish safety and trust, which are violently shaken.

Isolating secure support systems at work and home, people wrestle silently, overwhelmed by troubles too heavy to carry alone until their shoulders sag physically. Pride prevents them from admitting their struggles, despite depending on guidance to navigate challenges once easily conquered independently. A defeated aura trail marked by cynicism and apathy warns of sinking morale and threatening retention.

When punctuality, dress code, and meeting etiquette slip through the cracks, underlying exhaustion seeks shortcuts to finish seemingly impossible workloads. Attendance policies strain team commitments, relying on all contributors to be prepared. Quality and efficiency decline through chain reactions. Customer dissatisfaction spikes when neglected obligations pile up. Leaders who urged practicing self-care years ago to subordinate themselves, now model unhealthy extremes, warning just how far down gravity pulls before touching the bottom.

Thankfully, before hope extinguishes completely, reassessing brutal periods reframes stress as an unsustainable indicator of broken systems. Both resetting rhythms and restoring souls are needed. Healing happens through leaders courageously igniting cultural revolutions and rehumanizing work environments, one transparent conversation at a time.

Owning organizational shortfalls allows for authentic improvements, empowering staff to recapture purpose and passion. Some realignment means letting underperformers move on rather than prolonging bad fits for all. Consoling the remaining teams openly after layoffs builds trust for future flexibility. Clarifying work-from-home options accommodates family demands while affirming that output counts more than physical presence in the office.

Relieving excessive burdens reengages passion by reminding workers that their value exceeds productivity. Celebrate the devoted mentorship that shapes new hires. Compensate exceptional creative capital by reinvesting in continually bettering systems for all. Cheer on volunteering efforts, coordinating beloved holiday blood drives or summer sports teams. Link quarterly bonuses exceeding sales targets to local charities receiving grants.

When companies insist workers park their health and souls at the entry gates, dismissing humanity, innovation dulls over time. Restoring the rhythm begins with respecting employees' complex roles that balance beyond office walls. Nourish positive surprises through impromptu potlucks, flexible schedules, and purposeful collaborations. Productivity is grown through laughter, listening, and rediscovered self-expression. The future opens through loving people, not just chasing profits.

Strategies for Boosting Resilience and Balancing Professional Life

No one escapes work stresses completely—that's real life! But improving how we respond internally weakens their impacts, so we bounce back stronger. Building emotional muscles through a growth mindset, communication skills, and preventative self-care makes professional demands feel manageable, not crushing over the long haul. It takes discipline to consistently strengthen these resilience skills, but the payoff sustains careers and well-being through the inevitable storms ahead.

Choosing a growth mindset means we believe abilities keep developing rather than being fixed limitations. Through always learning on the job, we become adaptable, actually benefiting long-term from near-term failures, feedback, and setbacks that teach new perspectives. Maintaining teachability requires regulating ego and listening openly to colleagues with different experiences. Their unique insights enlighten creative solutions that are missed when tackling problems independently. Shared knowledge builds up faster, unlocking innovation and excellence that lifts teams collectively.

Emotional intelligence (EQ) distinguishes great leaders by empowering people through motivational vision and compassion. Self-awareness builds trust as you communicate transparently your personal strengths, blind spots, passions, and quirks. Modeling humility makes others feel safe admitting mistakes, knowledge gaps, and needing support. Leading vulnerably awakens loyalty beyond any fear-based boss. Managing anger and anxiety even amid uncertainty allows a non-anxious presence to immediately calm anxiety through grounded responsiveness. Empathizing emotionally before offering logical fixes makes others feel truly heard, understood, and valued.

Social connections energize workplace communities, overcoming isolation's exhaustion. Peer appreciation feeds accomplishment, recognizing progress on shared goals. Former teammates keep that advice and encouragement years later, cementing purposeful work. Quick check-ins without transactional urgency build rapport and connections beyond the surface level. Celebrating personal milestones like birthdays, pregnancies, or marathons humanizes through expressing care beyond projects alone. Even small talk about family or hobbies eases stress, reminding us that whole, complex individuals clock in daily, not productivity units.

Balancing professional demands with self-care prevents physical and emotional burnout. Regular preventative health habits like balanced nutrition, adequate sleep, and movement boost the immune system, cognitive focus, and a positive outlook, keeping up peak performance. Restorative practices like massages, spending time in nature, and uplifting hobbies relieve mental fatigue. Setting boundaries around work hours, notifications, and emotional investment establishes a healthy balance between multiple priorities. Decompressing through routines like mindfulness meditation or journaling clarifies overwhelming tasks. Ultimately, careers require a marathon mindset, not manic sprints risking rapid flameouts. Renewal keeps up in the long race by respecting human holistic needs.

Proactively managing expectations prevents last-minute crunches that overwhelm capacity repeatedly. Estimate project timelines; putting in extra time knowing that the unknown adds hidden delays and rework. Say no, responsibly ensuring excellence on agreed priorities rather than overpromising and struggling later to deliver. Delegate or outsource secondary items, preserving focus on the make-or-break goals only you can champion with savvy vision.

Honing problem-solving skills prepares you to respond amid uncertainties with flexible options. Break intimidating challenges into step-by-step plans that are easier to slowly influence. Consult mentors, researchers, and peers with specialized experience before finalizing strategies. Monitor progress, celebrating small milestones that build momentum. Embrace the process, knowing that a few solutions are perfectly smooth every time. Structure what-if contingency plans to ensure eagerly improving systems are ongoing.

Change in management depends on adaptability in transitioning projects or even whole companies amid shifts in market priorities over the years. Consider diverse insights before determining direction. Allow adjustments as new data emerges. Frame the next phase positively, honoring contributions from past seasons while inspiring progress. Migrate loyal teams gradually across mile markers through transparency, rationale, and empathy for their personal transitions in roles or job security.

Address building conflicts early before tensions erupt, fracturing relationships, or stalling projects. Hear all perspectives fully before reacting, finding shared truth from different angles. Differentiate opinion from facts, focusing on the issues and not attacking character. Apologize for the miscommunication and your contribution amid the misunderstanding. Seek solutions, prioritizing collective goals above ego. Follow up respectfully, ensuring a resolution, before resuming business as usual. Apply lessons learned to improve patterns going forward.

As boundaries blur between remote work and home demands, maintaining a healthy balance grows increasingly important yet challenging. Schedule focused blocks designated solely for completing deliverables without distraction from messages or meetings. Set automatic away messages on weekends, directing non-urgent contacts to when you return. Establish no-meeting timeslots for strategizing, remember that creative ideation flows best without interruption. Switch off notifications during family dinners or youth activities, honoring priorities beyond the office. Coworkers respecting your time signals that you equally respect theirs.

Even leaders perform better through ongoing input polished by accountability. Welcome critiques of proposals during brainstorming, strengthening vision before large-scale rollout. Seek metrics and anonymous surveys evaluating team support qualitatively and quantitatively. Feedback is the breakfast of champions committed to continual improvement.

With these tips in practice in the workplace, problems feel less oppressive. Recognize control lies in the chosen response, not the events themselves. Redirect what weighs personally toward action steps moving circumstances forward. Release anxiety around the vague through radical self-trust in timing and process. Storms eventually pass; resilient individuals and teams anchor their values regardless of external shakeups. You were made to weather every season, transforming challenges into growth.

Part 5:

Endurance and Longevity in Resilience

Chapter 10:
Emotional Armor—Building Resilience from the Inside Out

Navigating life's roughest rapids demands more than sheer brute force, and power-steering reactions downstream. Skillful self-awareness and inner compass clarity likewise determine which way we emerge from the whitewater crossroads. When cascading crises cloud vision for the best life path, strengthening emotional armor and buoyancy keep us afloat until moving waters calm.

Essentially, this means strategically growing emotional intelligence (EQ) to balance intellect—using awareness and wisdom about our humanity as much as external knowledge for solving modern problems. Honing navigation senses for reading warning ripples before overwhelming waves allows one to proactively prepare rather than desperately reacting when swept into distress unexpectedly.

Think of EQ resilience competencies in maritime terms: identifying damaging tidal triggers; crewing trusted community connections; mapping mental escape routes when floods rise; signaling SOS notices when temporarily overwhelmed; avoiding shame riptides; and ultimately guiding vessels toward calmer karma waters where growth flows.

The Role of Emotional Intelligence in Building Resilience

Emotions move as fast as whitewater rapids, often catching us off guard with changing intensities. Building resilience to handle unpredictable currents and hidden rocks demands equally agile skills for sensing undercurrents within. Just as radar guides pilots through storm turbulence, clarity on our emotional terrain maps routes to navigate life's twists and turns.

This self-perceptive ability is called emotional intelligence. Unlike IQ smarts gained through academics, EQ develops from repeatedly facing inner rumblings with courage rather than avoiding discomfort until overwhelmed. Reading your warning signs allows you to proactively prepare so crisis moments become growth catalysts rather than capsizing traps.

Emotional Intelligence Components

EQ includes five core sensing capabilities working together seamlessly once honed:

- **Self-awareness**: Self-awareness skills read our emotional radar screens accurately, tuning into anger sparks or joy surges without judgment, so they can pass through constructively. Noticing inner physical sensations, triggers, patterns, and stories reveals how we uniquely experience situations. Building this sensitivity prevents denial when challenges inevitably strike. We gain power by naming our experiences.

- **Self-regulation**: Next up, self-regulation capacities steady the helm when alarm systems reactively misread charts. This allows emotions to intensify without losing situational control or rational perspective. Grounding anxious nerves, uplifting deflated moods, and allowing for appropriate expression without suppressing them prevents over- or under-reacting. Building healthy regulation through lifestyle habits creates resilience reserves for weathering storms in a balanced state.

- **Motivation**: Meanwhile, motivational radars lock onto values and dreams, sparking inner drive and purpose. Envisioning those desired horizons channels energies into constructive priorities and actions despite obstacles or boredom spells trying to divert routes. Whether escaping toxicity, establishing security, or protecting relationships, internal clarity on the why makes the *how-to* flow smoothly when riding emotional rapids. Your inner compass knows the way, whatever external currents there are.

- **Empathy**: Empathy skills also enable resilient navigation by accurately feeling others' experiences, often differing radically from our own. This emotional intelligence prevents projection biases and opens creative solutions only visible through diverse viewpoints. Compassionate listening replaces assumptions over similarities, allowing collaboration even amid disagreement. Conflict resolution flows from empathic insight.

- **Social skills**: Finally, social skills complete EQ capacities by integrating self and others' awareness into positive collective experiences through vulnerability, play, or mutually fulfilling support. Building intimacy comes through courageously expressing needs while generously encouraging the strengths of others in tandem. The result is bonding buoyancy amid shared rapids. The community prevents isolation while providing fallback stability when individual boats wobble.

Resilience demands balancing self-care and situational clarity to interact smoothly with ever-changing environments and people. Understanding our emotional world—what makes us tick—allows us to effectively engage life's clockwork beyond just reactively trying to control everything futilely. Developing EQ aligns us to flow with changing tides by using awareness and agency together. Internal and external emotional radars together guide us onward!

Importance of Emotional Intelligence in Resilience Development

No one escapes dealing with floods of anger, anxiety, sadness, or stress in life—not even the Dalai Lama himself! The difference is whether or not emotional waves wash away stability as a result of catching us unaware and overwhelming our coping capacities fast. Building resilience to handle inner turbulence starts with reading the radar of your unique emotional terrain accurately, and then charting skillful responses ahead of time. Resilience rides on emotional intelligence!

The better we know our caution signs for Burnout Boulevard or Anxious Avenue, the sooner we take healthy detours by reaching out, restoring work-life balance, or practicing self-care. EQ prevents denial of losing direction or limiting beliefs that reduce power over inner experiences and reactions. It's life-saving psycho-navigation when facing modern challenges!

Let's break down key areas of emotional awareness and control to reduce pressure and prevent worse crises from brewing:

- EQ allows for catching overly intensive stress spikes before a physical and mental health nosedive. Identifying emotional exhaustion, irritability, concentration lapses, or escapist cravings early provides us the gift of pausing counterproductively excessive workloads and pulling triple overtime on empty. Preventing full flaming out preserves joie de vivre!

- Similarly, emotional self-checks notice emotional numbing, cynicism, or feelings of inadequacy or prolonged strain before hitting a heart attack pace. Reigniting work purpose and social connections counteracts classic burnout through renegotiated responsibilities that are aligned with authentic priorities. You can't pour from an empty cup!

- Beyond mitigating damage, EQ skills compound everyday satisfaction by clearly highlighting individual passions, talents, and meaning sources to direct choices. Understanding unique emotional needs shapes work-life synergies where careers and relationships energize rather than compete through draining compromise. It's about working smarter, not harder or longer!

- In that vein, self-aware people sidestep unhealthy habits, attempting to allow difficult emotions to pass by at the moment so they can be processed later, initiating healing. Smoking, overeating, overspending, or avoidance coping might offer temporary relief but compound long-term stress by masking growth opportunities. EQ allows constructively engaging vulnerability with courage rather than avoidance.

- Similarly, self-regulation prevents impulsive self-sabotage from intense feelings hijacking logical priorities at the moment. Short-term mood fixing often creates downstream obstacles, derailing resilience. Constructively riding emotional waves makes space for more empowered responses in the long term. No shame, just growth!

- The benefit is exponentially compounding positive progress from increasing emotional coherence with each small win. Ultimately, EQ cultivates reservoirs of resilience, purpose, and belonging, buffering against destructive urges when adversity strikes—exactly when needed most! It becomes easier and more automatic to bounce back the more practiced these skills become in everyday circumstances.

In essence, emotional awareness gifts internal guidance systems, protecting the resilience needed to weather external storms now and in the future. It may seem airy-fairy or touchy-feely, but statistically sharp EQ strongly correlates with tangible mental health, life satisfaction, and relationship harmony measures over time by preventing cycles of unnecessary suffering. That skill is utterly priceless!

Emotional Mastery

Choppy waters challenge every sailor, so grabbing that emotional steering wheel with both hands matters!

Self-Awareness

Self-awareness allows us to navigate feelings constructively, so we drive reactions rather than getting hijacked onto rocky shores. Beyond suppressing or venting frustrations reflexively, insight guides responses aligned with inner truth. Let's break down practical steps using the rooted mindfulness movement (RAIN) system for building emotional mastery from the inside out!

RAIN simply offers a mental checklist recognizing inner experiences, allowing space for their intensity, investigating with non-judgmental curiosity, and preventing identity fusion so emotions don't define your entirety.

Recognition means tuning into physical sensations, images, self-talk stories, or impulses arising in reaction to people or events, internally or externally. Maybe muscle tension, resurfacing memories, racing thoughts, or irritation emerge. The key is gently noticing signals without analyzing the reasons behind them or leaping into problem-solving just yet. Stay open and present with the feeling at first, rather than dismissing irritability by downplaying its validity. Allow the emotion its due space, even if it seems irrational later. Suppressing rarely helps in the long run!

Once aware of an emotion swelling internally, pause strategically to allow its natural wave to crest and fall without fueling unnecessary intensity. Breathe slowly while labeling the core sensation without second-guessing causes or questioning its legitimacy based on outside opinions. Stay grounded in your own direct experience for clarity! This prevents preemptive reactions while response options expand.

Next, investigate the unfolding experience with open curiosity, not clouded by self-judgment or defensiveness, once heightened intensity settles. What personal interpretations, memories, or urges activate alongside the core sadness, anger, or insecurity itself? How specifically does this feeling manifest uniquely for you—physically, behaviorally, or narratively? What new self-understanding emerges from befriending rather than battling perceived negativity flooding your system? Insight rises by diving in, not avoiding!

Finally, prevent fusing personal identity wholly with emotions inevitably passing through based on circumstances or biochemistry rather than self-worth. Saying, "I feel rage" versus "I am enraged" allows us to see the layers of experience in emotions. Noticing feelings as temporary states rather than permanent traits creates freedom in adjusting behaviors accordingly without inner self-blame too! This builds agency by responding wisely as needed in the moment.

Cultivating RAIN skills forms the bedrock of resilience, which is made of emotional literacy, responsive flexibility, and self-leadership. But consistent practice makes perfect; hence, tools for expanding self-oriented awareness help drive change. Start unlocking your EQ potential!

Keep an ongoing journal, tracking feelings, triggers, reactions, and evolving patterns over time. Writing regularly builds tangible fluency, identifying and articulating your emotional terrain with nuance so it feels familiar. Progress, not perfection, counts here, so don't filter for polished prose or impactful insights right away. Raw reality offers the richest material, revealing unconscious inner workings!

Schedule occasional mindfulness sessions for intentional scanning of your mental, emotional, and physical landscapes without any particular goal beyond non-judgmental noticing. Tune into sensations, moods, self-talk tendencies, or subtle behavior shifts across various activities. Curiosity about the vibrant complexity within cultivates compassion and insight into shared human experiences, uniting us all! Every life holds beauty and pain.

Weaving self-oriented questions into routine conversations likewise builds emotional awareness and fitness. How am I interpreting this situation emotionally? How might other perspectives exist beyond my own? What past experiences shape my reactions now? How might I reframe my response for more empowering outcomes? Am I projecting exhaustion or anxiety negatively without evidence? Keep it real and productive!

Speaking uplifting truths aloud daily rewires critical neural pathways, prioritizing self-growth over habitual judgment in society's relentless competition. Even two minutes of sincerely praising efforts, envisioning positive outcomes, or expressing gratitude for challenges forcing growth makes space for resilience in the long run. Affirmations make way for actualization; try it!

Enlightening emotional awareness takes commitment but delivers essential clarity and agency for constructively relating with the world. The time is now for each of us to bravely harness an understanding of the only heart truly in our hands—our own.

Self-Regulation

Emotions naturally ebb and flow like the tides—often intensely, whether we approve logically or not. Attempting to suppress normal reactions causes more harm than good in the long run. Like forcing waves backward ultimately creates a tsunami, blocking vulnerable feelings builds pressure guaranteed to erupt later!

Emotional flexibility preserves health and relationships far better over time compared to rigid stoicism or volatility. Building resilience depends on riding the emotional waves skillfully with protective gear when needed, rather than avoiding water altogether. This emotional mastery ability is called self-regulation; let's dive into how it works!

Attention basics set the stage by carefully monitoring internal experiences with radar-like precision but without immediate reaction. Noticing physical cues, uncomfortable thoughts, building frustration, or a deflated mood prevents being blindsided when bigger feelings suddenly swell and spill over. Rational effectiveness depends partly on reading warning signs early before losing situational awareness.

Acceptance also allows for making space for the reality of occasionally messy emotions recognizing them as normal and biologically intended reactions rather than threats to control at all costs. Despite cultural messaging that unwavering happiness equals success, even Disney characters and the many Dalai Lamas inevitably experience anger, anxiety, grief, guilt, and doubt! Denying core humanity causes more harm than help when genuinely striving for resilience.

Expecting emotions does not mean endlessly venting without accountability. Like the focused power of rivers or waves, feelings contain energy for potential constructive use, not just reckless devastation. Emotional intelligence means learning to harness intense reactions for cathartic insight, creative breakthroughs, vulnerability when bonding with others, or driving toward meaningful purposes beyond simply following rash impulses alone.

For example, anger often signals important boundaries being crossed, which now deserve loving communication, either externally or internally. Hurt underpins anger once those righteous flames cool to embers—then fresh opportunities emerge from working collaboratively. New emotional wisdom prevents future crossed wires through updated policies or habits.

Similarly, anxiety or envy contain clues to self-limiting stories that secretly erode the confidence needed for reaching goals or voicing overlooked needs, causing resentment. Reframing self-talk into empowering perspectives allows oneself to move positively ahead, no longer chained to past measures. The light gets brighter by turning inward for truth.

Even grief, a loved one's final gift, brings the heart closer through remembrance and gratitude. This stays with us until joy returns, renewed by timeless bonds. More things grow in the garden when certain plants pass on. Rumi's immortal wisdom reveals to us this nugget of truth.

Of course, until emotionally attuned regulation skills develop through consistent practice, additional backup tools in the resilience toolkit assist in staying grounded when flooded by emotions. Physical movement, casual conversations, creative immersion, or timeout space all temporarily reduce intensity so higher logic can regain the wheel. There is no shame in using guardrails when needed!

Building individual emotional muscles also prevents overburdening relationships unfairly, allowing more space for mutual support. Setting healthy boundaries means acknowledging personal self-care needs and collective moral duties without martyring one for the other in the long term. Balanced Equity sustains positive bonds and communities.

Over time, with compassionate commitment, emotional rollercoasters smooth into wavelengths where the presence of the mind connects to the presence of the heart. This fusion empowers responding gracefully to whatever arises within or without. Serenity emerges when fighting no longer remains.

In essence, radical self-acceptance soothes struggles by removing the judgment that healing somehow equals weakness. Life offers experiences to grow empathy and deepen purpose. Each feeling, no matter how disruptive in the moment, serves this benefit when given spacious reverence.

Motivation

Stress is unavoidable, but getting stuck in crisis mode is optional as long as we keep moving forward bit by bit. Motivation fuels that progress when adversity and exhaustion make surrender appealing. With emotional intelligence guiding the inner compass toward a purpose beyond momentary moods, we can navigate with resilience, flowing more smoothly without losing hope. Let's map out how to stay on course in stormy seas!

Goal setting primes motivation best when framed realistically for your current tools and temperament. Getting clear on the emotional *why* behind desired outcomes builds organic drive better than shouldering unrealistic expectations. These unrealistic expectations are bound to cause us to crumble midstream under their weight—then drive and perseverance wash away. Small, consistent targets encourage action and progress, building emotional muscles over time through incremental success.

For example, shy Katy dreaded job interviews, triggering the trauma and self-doubt associated with memories of past rejections. Rather than demanding she power through paralyzing anxiety overnight, she broke the process into step-by-step emotional training goals: first practicing deep breathing relaxation when simply imagining interviews; then roleplaying introductions with a supportive friend to understand her competence in the situation. These small emotional achievements fueled confidence in larger conversations later. Before long, Katy sailed smoothly through multiple job interviews with resilience!

Like exercising a healing muscle gradually so it strengthens without strain, pace emotional expansion challenges just slightly beyond your current capability—without overextending abilities that are bound to rupture and require restarting. Patience prevents undermining progress through perfectionism that punishes rather than encourages. Trust in the process!

That said, resist complacency by adding a slight additional tension regularly. This will help grow new emotional membranes instead of having rigid walls that attempt to block adversity altogether. If no tears mean no gain, then truly tears mean terrain for reinforcing worthy skills.

Some fears may persist, yet still find footing with time by leaning into motivation for meaningful horizons ahead.

For example, Seema knew her quick defensive reactions prevented vulnerable intimacy in relationships. Rather than attacking herself as emotionally broken, she reframed sensitivity as strength warranting protection when honored, not hidden. This self-permission allowed gradually requesting partners to pause disputes, initiating constructive dialogs about underlying feelings later when calm. Emotional risks sustain confidence in asking for healthy needs in the long run.

Regardless of the domain, maintain resilience momentum by routinely celebrating small signals of positive direction, through journaling gratitude, self-praise, or creative expression. Even ordinary home chores or unglamorous tasks deserve applause if completing them fuels personal progress and emotional well-being. Completing a week without social media or courageously candid conversation is an immense emotional achievement, though subtle externally. Build up your credibility with consistency to expand comfort zones incrementally yet sustainably. What we water, blooms within over time.

Remember that falling short or hitting obstacles signals only momentary roadblocks along much longer journeys if determined vision persists flexibly. Breathe through the discomfort, get creative, find alternate pathways, and lean on support systems to renew emotional reserves depleted midstream. These ups and downs inevitably arise for everyone in all endeavors, and understanding this means frustration becomes merely feedback. By working through initial frustration, the next wise action toward destiny is revealed.

In many ways, emotional intelligence builds like physical health—through consistent, compassionate care rather than sporadic aggressive pushes followed by breakdown and abandonment cycles because they are too hard. Remain mindful of realistic bandwidth goals while still seeking meaningful progress through incremental input raised over time. With understanding and kindness, motivation fuels whatever arises!

Empathy

Connecting with others means genuinely hearing and sitting with their often vastly different experiences without dismissing them as exaggerated, understated, or attempting fast fixes. Compassion arises first by making space for struggle through listening ears, open minds, and kind hearts. Judgment predicts while empathy comprehends. Let's explore habits that welcome authentic emotional exchanges!

Start by simply allowing people full freedom to express themselves without interruption. Concentrate completely on their words and unspoken feelings conveyed through facial cues, gestures, and tone fluctuations. Let their unfolding narrative flow like music as understanding builds, before considering your replies or reactions. Patience allows the truth to emerge.

When confused, gently dig deeper through curious questions, exploring the context and meanings you may have missed. Seek clarifying examples if descriptions seem unclear. Reflect on what you heard in your own words to confirm you have accurately captured their perspectives and associated emotions. Accuracy confirms the safety of sharing vulnerably.

Equally importantly, catch the impulse to dismiss others' differing takes by hastily reassuring them not to worry or feel upset. The fact is, they do worry and feel upset—for good reasons, making sense in their shoes! The goal becomes not fixing discomfort but demonstrating presence with it. Shared struggles bond more than surface cheerfulness alone. Create space for the truth.

Consider openly sharing occasions when you also wrestled with similar emotions or situations yourself, made mistakes handling them initially, or how you are still learning. This vulnerability normalizes such adversity as something everyone experiences over time. Revealing fallibility by example encourages courage and comfort in unpacking suppressed struggles, as others often hide their struggles silently and alone. Your vulnerability allows them an opportunity to vent.

For extra empathy insight, purposefully surround yourself with diverse people and perspectives beyond the habitual echo chambers of those mirroring similar limitations or advantages as your own. Whether through books, films, friends, or volunteer work, exposure to unfamiliar people and ideas expands mental and emotional mobility, identifying common resilience barriers faced by wider communities. Point your gaze inward through outward windows!

Speaking of volunteering, get involved with local organizations or causes empowering those overcoming struggles, such as homelessness, disability discrimination, domestic violence aftermath, or grief support groups. Offer practical help or simply listen to those trusting your compassion. Such humility profoundly awakens gratitude and empathy, even amid your unresolved trials. We rise together.

Practice embodied emotional sensing through body-centered mindfulness meditations. Scan for physical sensations manifesting when recalling arguments, receiving criticism, or facing uncertainty. Recognize these biological reactions as value-neutral indicators of humanity's shared vulnerability. Giving a physical dimension to emotional experiences builds intuitive clarity around common triggers, understandable reactions, and pathways holding space for mutual understanding. The sacred lives within all life's emotions.

The bottom line remains to honor each person's right to determine their emotional reality. Judging who should feel what denies fundamental dignity. Deep listening and suspended assumptions make way for trust, truthful expression, and conflict resolution. More divides people than emotions themselves; we all want happiness, love, and peace at our core. Lead first with the heart through empathy.

Social Skills

Having strong social skills allows you to interact positively with others in personal and professional settings. Some helpful strategies include:

- **listen**: Focus fully on the person talking without interrupting. Look them in the eyes, nod sometimes, and ask good questions to show you care about what they say. Don't let things around you or your thoughts distract you. That way, the other person will feel heard, and you may even see that you find what they say interesting.

- **Communicate clearly**: Speak audibly, with proper enunciation so you are easily understood. Use vocabulary suitable for the situation. Be concise yet descriptive. A chance to ask clarifying questions should be given to the other individual.

- **Show interest in others**: Have good discussions where everyone can share. Ask questions that let people tell you more than just yes or no. Make sure others feel comfortable opening up about their ideas, life experiences, and interests, even if they don't agree with you. Give them your full attention and recognize different views as equally valid, so they feel respected when talking with you. Keep conversations two-way by letting others speak as much as you do.

- **Enhance verbal and non-verbal cues**: Mind both what you say and how you say it. Modulate tone, volume, and inflection to convey appropriate emotion. Similarly, use positive body language like smiling, facing the person, and maintaining an open posture. Ensure your words and body work in harmony.

- **Listen to feedback**: Be receptive to constructive criticism and guidance. Do not get defensive; truly consider the message. Implement suggested improvements with an open mind, viewing feedback as an opportunity for personal growth. Thank the person for caring enough to share their insight with you.

- **Observe social skills in action**: Notice how those who are skilled at interacting with others navigate conversations, demonstrate care and inclusiveness, and resolve differences respectfully. Reflect on behaviors you may wish to integrate into your style. We continue learning our whole lives by remaining curious and humble.

- **Practice confident eye contact**: Look directly at the speaker rather than down or around. Do not stare intensely, but connect genuinely through the eyes. This builds trust and attentiveness. Break contact briefly on occasion before reciprocating again. With close friends, eye contact can communicate support during difficult conversations.

- **Ask open-ended questions**: Inquire about subjects that require detailed responses: "What goals are you prioritizing this year and how can I help support you?" rather than "Do you have any goals this year?" Open-ended questions drive substantive discussions by urging the speaker to provide meaningful elaboration.

- **Develop icebreaker questions**: Have some go-to questions in your back pocket to initiate interactions: "What is the most interesting thing you have read lately?" or "If you could travel anywhere in the world, where would you go?" Icebreakers jumpstart fulfilling conversations by introducing novel, fun topics.

Implementing even a few of these tips can vastly strengthen social skills, enrich relationships, and improve well-being. Of course, navigating interpersonal relationships requires ongoing practice. Be patient with yourself and others. By gradually building emotional mastery, you can have healthier, more rewarding connections.

Path to Positivity

Even when times are tough, it helps to stay positive. Looking on the bright side makes us stronger, so we can handle whatever life throws our way. People who are usually upbeat tend to be less stressed and healthier overall. They're also happier with how things turn out. Feeling joy, love, wonder, motivation, pride in your accomplishments, humor, and curiosity is good for your growth as a person. These positive emotions lead to gaining wisdom and feeling your best, both mentally and physically. Positive emotions hold the keys to improving your well-being.

We all have access to positive emotions, though some may come more naturally to particular personalities. Regardless of our tendencies, there are actions we can take to foster pleasant feelings and lift our spirits. Simple daily habits can nurture emotional wellness.

Practice Gratitude

Take a few quiet moments to reflect on the people and things you appreciate, big or small. This might be family, friends, health, favorite foods, music you love, positive memories, acts of kindness from others, and so on. Verbalize the gratitude or write a thank-you note when possible.

Stay in the Present

Rather than dwelling on the past or worrying about the future, bring attention to the gift that is this very moment, right here, right now. Notice your surroundings using all five senses or focus on tasks without judgment. This mindfulness keeps us grounded in positivity.

Engage in Uplifting Activities

Choose hobbies and pastimes that spark joy. Some examples are listening or dancing to lively music, exploring inspiring nature settings, playing with beloved pets, engaging in stimulating conversations, reading novels or poetry, photography, journaling, or viewing or creating any art form that elicits an emotional lift.

Cultivate Positive Emotions

Just as we can strengthen muscles with focused effort, we can train our brains to produce pleasant emotions more readily through regular practice. Think of hope, inspiration, calm, interest, pride, amusement, and awe. What brings you these feelings? Set the intention each day to tap into positivity through thoughts, language, behaviors, and exposure to elevating stimuli like music or comedy.

Take Care of Physical Health

Our mental and emotional states are intricately connected with our bodily condition. Ensure adequate, restful sleep and nutrition from healthy, energizing foods. Exercise elevates mood while also keeping the body fit. Manage stress levels through sufficient relaxation. A healthy organism fosters positivity.

Find Purpose and Meaning

Identify the core values that give your life meaning: family, faith, learning, creativity, community service, ethics, and so on. Set goals aligned with your sense of purpose around career, relationships, personal growth, hobbies, health, or other areas providing fulfillment. Discover and activate your passions!

Develop Healthy Physical Habits

Our physical condition profoundly impacts our emotions. Ensure adequate, restful sleep to wake up refreshed. Incorporate nutritious whole foods like fruits, veggies, lean proteins, and healthy fats to stabilize energy and moods. Stay hydrated and limit sugar and caffeine. Movement is key—walk, stretch, dance, play sports, and strength train. Getting outdoors boosts positivity!

Practice Mindfulness and Relaxation

Stress and worrying about the future or past deplete pleasant emotions. Mindfulness keeps us grounded in the present moment, the only place we have power. Relaxation techniques also help release unwanted tension. Consider:

- **Breath Focus**: Sit comfortably with eyes closed and bring full attention to inhales and exhales. Place one hand on the belly and one on the chest, feeling the air fill the lungs. Count breaths or say "in" and "out" silently. Even one minute of conscious breathing induces calm.
- **Body scan**: Systematically notice physical sensations in each body part without judging discomfort. Release tension with each

long exhale, relaxing muscles bit by bit until reaching a deeply soothed state. This practice requires staying present.

- **Meditation**: Sit upright in a serene space. Breathe naturally and return focus to the present each time the mind wanders. Thoughts and feelings will come and go, but remain anchored and observe them without attachment. This creates mental and emotional balance.

- **Guided imagery**: Listen to a recording that leads you through envisioning a peaceful scene like lying in soft grass watching clouds drift by. The goal is to feel immersed using all five senses. This transports our consciousness to serene places.

- **Mind-body practices**: Yoga, tai chi, and qigong unite breath, movement, and stillness to relax and build awareness of how mental states influence the physical being. Choose beginner-level sessions to avoid strain. End with a resting pose.

- **Repetitive prayer**: Those with spiritual inclinations may find that centering prayer or mantra repetition channels awareness toward the sacred, activating faith to evoke comforting states of peace, love, and hope. Welcome any emotions arising.

Set Small Goals

Structure activities into achievable steps. Give yourself credit for all progress to activate pride and motivation for the next step. Goals provide direction and bolster self-confidence as we check off accomplishments.

By actively and consistently focusing on gratitude, presence, uplifting activities, emotional development, and physical and mental self-care, we chart an empowering path to positivity. Mindset is a powerful tool. Our lens shapes our reality. Deliberately fostering positive emotions builds resilience to adversity and amplifies joy, benefiting yourself and the community. What steps will you take today toward greater emotional well-being?

We each hold the capacity for positivity and calm, even amid chaos. By devoting focus and time to purpose, holistic self-care, and present-moment awareness, we summon these emotional resources, and they strengthen with ongoing practice. What uplifting ritual shall you integrate today?

Chapter 11:

Stand Strong in the Storm—Enhancing Resilience in Times of Crisis

Few scenarios test our mettle and mental strength more intensely than an unanticipated crisis. Disaster our lives apart, from comforting calm into chaos This storm pushes fears, anxiety, and desperation onto us when reliable foundations crumble unexpectedly. Whether it is personal pain or global events devastating communities, crises signal uncertainty suddenly as new harsh realities enter our lives overnight. Survival instincts push systems into hypervigilance, trying to steady boats amid harrowing storms no one saw gathering on horizons now flooded by harsh waves.

In these turbulent times, resilience becomes lifesaving to prevent drowning amid dangers and change. People working through traumatic disasters share common strategies for strengthening their capacity to withstand hardship. Their game plans offer valuable crisis management skills that prepare and empower all of us to become more consciously crisis-ready through building resilience skills over time. Then, when the crisis enters our lives, emotional muscles and memory kick in to guide teams safely onto higher ground again.

No one withstands trauma completely unshaken at the core. Grief must be given space alongside caring for urgent matters needing clear-headed action simultaneously. So, we'll talk through navigating emotional minefields while dealing with already pressing conditions made worse when neglected or denied. Strategic planning empowers quicker adaptability as conditions shift rapidly. But exhaustively mapping every detail also gives the false idea of total control, which can be harmful when certain variables escalate chaotically beyond our prediction. Wrestling fears bravely prevent inaction, while radical self-trust grows faith, building strength sufficient to face each wave without worrying about endless hypotheticals. Survival is possible, though the path weaves through narrow ledges, ones we may have thought impossible to cross in times of normalcy. As they say, "Where there is life, there is hope."

We hear story after story about how everyday heroes discovered power they never expected they had, holding space for others to unravel beside them. Trauma bonds people frequently, forging deep companionship growing past many former surface bonds once tying communities. Triumph often flows through relentless rivers of tears. Those who stood at the end of chaotic times victorious first had to stare demons in the face, refusing to hide away. Resilient individuals bend and adapt rather than snapping quickly. Crises reveal who shines brightest when the night seems darkest. And from the ashes, stars emerge even brighter, having grown to endure what few souls will ever endure in multiple lifetimes.

While no strategy substitutes fully for safety when crises escalate dangerously, those taking responsibility seriously listen to wisdom. They gather storm provisions and protective infrastructure to minimize harm from the forces of crisis. Your lifeboat was designed for choppy and rough waters, even if you are comfortable cruising calmer paths. Have faith in your ability to deal with adversity, trust in reliable companions navigating unpredictability, and awaken the courage to engage passionately nonetheless. How we make it through storms proves who we are when the skies eventually clear. You were made to weather floods and thrive—believe it.

Understanding Crisis Challenges and Emergencies

Few events shake life's foundations as abruptly as an unforeseen crisis, catapulting us into dizzying chaos immediately. Like power grids crashing regionally or news of sudden deaths upending families, disaster plunges everything familiar into unfamiliar panic, flooding rational thought. Survival instincts kick in, trying to maintain balance in a time of uncertainty.

By definition, a crisis is an unstable or crucial time when a difficult or important decision must be made with stakes running high. The Chinese character for crisis even combines the characters of danger and opportunity, reminding us that growth springs from important trials. While taxing mentally, physically, and emotionally as stability cracks, navigating deep crises ultimately strengthens those courageous enough to find meaning in the mess. Essentially, earthquakes reveal the integrity of infrastructure, preventing collapse. Resilience skills bear fruit solely through hardship. Calm seas never force skillful navigation against storms, which is why resilience can only come into play during times of hardship.

Catastrophes come in all shapes, from personal health emergencies or family disasters to widescale natural disasters, destroying entire cities suddenly and without mercy. Financial crashes liquidate wealth, building up over generations seemingly overnight. Hurricanes whiteout visibility, ripping roofs and roads up while loved ones scatter, evacuating hastily. Medical diagnoses like cancer, comas, or dementia rewrite once predictable futures, now hinging on variables no one can accurately predict. Even individual job losses or divorces unravel the primary pillars of identity, security, and community once seen as certain.

Amid such chaos, shock, and denial often accompany our first attempts at grasping this frightening new reality. Stress skyrockets when trying to deal with nonstop demands, changes by the minute, and exhaustion from relentless adaptation. Fear and anxiety grow against the overwhelming unknowns endlessly ahead. Trauma readily ambushes bodies and minds exhausted by relentless intensity, ruining rest. Critical problems jeopardize safety when responsibilities grow past anyone's former scope and preparation. What basic capacities could comfortably handle getting buried by skyscrapers of concern? Relief remains a distant mirage through a marathon of focus, requiring us to put our all into providing help which barely keeps heads bobbing above violently churning waters.

Over long periods, such intensity eats away at resilience reserves much quicker without equal time for intentional recovery. Adrenaline peaks then crashes, plummeting our mood, health, and judgment without caring support. Core pillars of identity, family, and purpose seem cut off from us, a new environment replacing all that was once beloved. Future dreams no longer align with the present, crises summoning heroic strength just to survive, hour to battered hour. Financial stability disappears overnight through disastrous healthcare costs and demolished homes. Possessions holding precious memories are destroyed. The community scatters to safety, relocating in a rush without the capacity to reconnect. No one escapes unrattled, watching stability and security disappear virtually instantly. People scramble for survival trying to save pieces of their lives from the rising destruction surrounding them uncontrollably. No one knows how long aftershocks will echo through their life as they try to rebuild post-trauma. But resilience is the one thing that can help navigate the necessary marathon of recovering from catastrophe's blows.

Resilience Guidance for Stressful Times

Hard times and stressful situations can feel tough and make us want to give up. It's natural to want to step back when facing challenges or sadness. However, we can improve our capacity to overcome obstacles and increase our adaptability in constructive ways. It is a strength that comes from building resilience. We can roll with the punches of life and endure difficult situations without breaking down if we possess resilience. Moreover, it implies that we are capable of growing stronger. Even when problems come, we have the power within us to carry on. To build resilience, we can learn coping skills. Then, when trouble strikes, we will have the tools to not just survive the hard times but to feel okay and keep moving forward. Resilience helps us live through tough periods in better shape than before.

Stage 1: Survive

In extremely difficult or traumatic situations, the first priority is to stabilize ourselves just enough to survive. Practicing extreme self-care and leveraging our relationships to get the support we vitally need.

- **Practice acceptance**: The first step in building resilience is to fully accept the reality of the difficult situation, rather than denying it or struggling against a new normal that is out of our control. Fighting what's already happened will only exhaust our limited emotional resources. Radical acceptance allows us to channel those resources into coping as constructively as possible.

- **Accept your feelings**: Hand in hand with the situation, acceptance is allowing ourselves to accept and express whatever emotions arise in response to difficulty or loss. Give yourself permission to grieve, yell, cry—whatever you authentically feel. Avoid suppressing natural reactions.

- **Reach out to others**: Isolation only makes stressful situations feel more overwhelming. Connection is critical. Even reaching out briefly via text, email, or call serves as a lifeline to anchor us to stable support. Prioritize nurturing relationships and spending time with a compassionate, caring company.

- **Don't withdraw**: When we feel overwhelmed already, the natural response is to withdraw further, often when the connection is needed most. Fight the urge to isolate. Stay engaged with supportive friends and family. Keep the channels open.

Stage 2: Adapt

As the initial intensity of the situation begins to pass, the focus shifts to adapting ourselves mentally, emotionally, and situationally to a new normal.

- **Expand your network**: Seek new connections—friends, communities, and organizations offering new perspectives and resources on adjusting to evolving circumstances.

- **Avoid negative people**: Limit interactions with consistently pessimistic or drama-creating personalities. They can strain already low mental and emotional reserves.

- **Invest in self-care**: Difficult transitions mean we must intentionally prioritize activities that soothe, nourish, and recover stressed minds and bodies—comfort foods, baths, naps, walks in nature, reading uplifting books, and many more.

Stage 3: Recover

As adaptation progresses, our most important task shifts to proactive recovery and healing residual trauma from the experience. Intentionally retraining thought patterns allows us to regain emotional and mental balance.

- **Look for meaning and purpose**: However seemingly unfair or senseless adversity can seem, actively looking for meaning in suffering often illuminates unexpected significance. The experience served a purpose and brought unforeseen gifts—strength and insight, for example. Looking for meaning provides reassurance that nothing is wasted.

- **Give help to others**: Reaching out to support others struggling with similar situations softens trauma's hard edges. Compassionate acts and service create gentler mindsets, benefiting both the giver and the receiver.

- **Pursue hobbies and interests**: Immersing ourselves in nourishing activities unrelated to trauma or loss directly builds the mental resilience to move forward. Give creative passions or long-neglected interests attention.

- **Stay motivated**: In adversity's aftermath, inaction, and lingering depression can stall progress. Combat this with vision boards, motivational media, accountability partners, or coaches to stay on track toward recovery-oriented goals.

- **Deal with problems—one step at a time**: Break the big, complex problems stemming from the trauma into manageable pieces. Like eating an elephant—one bite at a time. Tiny actions add up to substantial change over time.

Stage 4: Thrive

Leverage lessons and strengths learned through adversity to grow forward from the past, reaching boldly toward a new horizon. Position both yourself and others impacted to ultimately thrive at higher levels in the aftermath of a crisis.

Notice and actively celebrate small achievements and milestones in the recovery process, such as completing a walk around the block after an illness. Such wins build essential momentum.

By proactively strengthening our capacity for resilience using these techniques, we prepare ourselves to ride out life's inevitable storms. Strengthening mental, emotional, and social skills before adversity strikes prepares us for the challenges ahead. We can feel empowered knowing we've developed the resources to survive and recover stronger than before. What emerges is a finely-tuned ability to adapt to circumstances, find meaning in suffering, and ultimately thrive—not despite hardship but because of it.

Identifying Emotions During Crises

When we find ourselves amid a crisis event or traumatic situation such as a natural disaster, pandemic, accident, assault, sudden loss, or other adversity, we will inevitably experience a broad spectrum of thoughts, feelings, and physical reactions over which we initially have little control. Understanding the typical range of cognitive, emotional, physical, and behavioral responses during severely stressful circumstances allows us to normalize our experience instead of covering up initial panic over our reactions with shame, frustration, or isolation. Just remember: nearly all initial reactions are temporary, and do not define you as mentally weak or permanently broken.

Cognitive Reactions

- **Confusion and difficulty concentrating**: Your ability to focus, think clearly, or make sense of situational details can momentarily weaken without warning. Sudden confusion is normal. Don't panic. Breathe slowly. The fog will pass.

- **Difficulty making decisions**: Second-guessing choices or freezing when choices arise is common early in crises when our brains enter self-protective fight-flight-or-freeze mode. Give yourself grace rather than demanding impossible clarity.

- **Decreased alertness**: You may zone out frequently, misplace belongings, or lose track of time or obligations. Trauma hijacks the thinking centers of our brain—temporarily decreasing alertness is the natural result. Help counter it by getting extra rest, writing things down, and confirming appointments and tasks with text alerts or calendars.

- **Memory lapses**: Forgetfulness spikes during crises. Our minds protect us by moving energy away from non-essential functions like solid memory formation, so we can just handle the survival needs of the moment. Like awake dreaming, memory lapses will pass. To help in the moment, write down key information for future reference.

- **Frequent thoughts of the event**: Intrusive visions of the experience flooding your mind against your will and periodic thoughts on the crisis entering your mind are textbook normal. Breathe, stretch, or engage your senses to gently shift focus to the present. The mind will ease out thoughts about the situation with support over time.

Emotional Reactions

- **Anger**: Irritability, misdirected frustration, and anger often emerge strongly post-crisis, triggered by feelings of vulnerability and grief. Punch pillows, stomp, or expend pent-up physical and emotional energy in safe bursts. Remind yourself that your feelings will shift.

- **Anxiety**: Panic attacks, constant worry, worst-case scenario thinking, and even intense, specific fears crop up due to nervous system overload. Use calming apps, stretch, and breathe slowly. Anxiety always passes if we don't buy into our thoughts as permanent realities.

- **Depression**: Hopelessness, profound sadness, and a lack of motivation or enjoyment in normal activities can arise and linger after tragic events. If persisting beyond a few weeks, seek counseling support. Temporary depressive symptoms are expected. You do not have a forever-defective personality now. Light will return.

- **Emotional numbness**: In contrast, some initially feel void of any emotion following a crisis—autopilot takes over because feeling anything seems impossible. Dissociative numbness shields us when sensations get too intense. Don't shame numbness. Slowly, feelings will unfold at a pace you can handle better.

- **Apathy or boredom**: Also common is a lack of interest, emotion, or the ability to feel concerned about anything. Activities normally enjoyed feel meaningless. The apparent boredom helps us retreat and save resources for future use. It's not permanent, and engagement will organically renew. Don't demand it prematurely.

- **Frustration**: Irritability from a lack of perceived control and feeling limited in supporting roles we value can certainly create frequent frustration post-crisis. Allow yourself to feel anger or even jealousy over others' unaffected lives. Nature designed frustration to encourage change. Use it proactively when possible.

Physical Reactions

- **Fatigue**: The crisis likely took massive physical, mental, and emotional energy from you, increasing your fight-or-flight hormones for a time. Afterward, profound fatigue sets in from the withdrawal of these stimulating chemicals, much like an adrenaline hangover. Nap when possible. Accept that you will be far more tired than usual for a while—it's nature's way of forcing us to physically rest while processing trauma.

- **Insomnia**: Alternatively, constant anxiety may translate into severe insomnia and an inability to relax into sleep despite utter exhaustion. Do not worry; it is normal. Maintain sleep hygiene rhythms and speak to a doctor if poor sleep continues for more than two weeks.

- **Headaches**: High blood pressure and clenched muscles from constant stress commonly cause headaches—sometimes even migraines—due to inflammation pathways activated by trauma. Over-the-counter pain relief, warm showers, calming walks outdoors, and rest often help ease pain.

- **Nausea and gastrointestinal problems**: Digestive issues are universally common post-crisis. Slow stomach emptying, diarrhea, or total appetite loss from excess stress hormones impacting smooth muscle function in the gut frequently create gastric distress. Drink fluids, eat smaller meals, and minimize the intake of inflammatory foods.

- **Hunger or loss of appetite**: The crisis may have suppressed appetite, but pent-up cortisol and fight-or-flight hormones eventually surge, driving excessive hunger for comfort foods. Persistent stress could eliminate appetite in post-crisis depression. Honor genuine cravings and nourish yourself. Eat only when truly hungry, and stop when full. Appetite will self-regulate later.

Behavioral Reactions

- **Withdrawal from others**: Don't panic if your natural tendency post-crisis becomes avoiding calls and missing events even from close loved ones. We often retreat socially while trauma settles subconsciously. Limit time alone if solitude reinforces depressive thoughts. Small talk is okay initially. Follow cues welcoming deeper discussion only when authentically ready.

- **Restlessness**: Pacing, agitation, and physical restlessness frequently emerge as products of free-floating anxiety or a burst of crisis-triggered fight-or-flight adrenaline, all looking for an outlet. Allow yourself constructive physical release without judgment. Safe, intense exercise, loud music, and stomping can help bleed off nervous energy productively.

- **Hypervigilance**: You may notice startling reactions, scanning crowds for danger, obsessively checking locks, or an inability to sit with your back exposed. Trauma automatically wires us into a higher level of self-protection mode temporarily. Ease slowly out of hypervigilance, sleeping with lights on if needed, and reminding yourself you are safe now.

- **Blaming others**: Strong urges to unfairly blame family, authorities, God, or random individuals for perceived preventable harm or inadequate crisis response often crop up post-trauma. Aim anger instead at the actual people responsible or faulty systems, if possible. Either way, progress lies in letting go of blame over time.

- **Substance abuse**: Reaching for substances to numb emotional or physical reactions is extremely common following tragedy. But it often reinforces depressive tendencies. While brief medications can help stabilize sleep, anxiety, or pain symptoms, address root causes through counseling and support groups as soon as you're ready.

By recognizing these responses as very normal following something abnormal and traumatic, we can begin accepting and addressing reactions properly. But remind loved ones also that while crisis reactions feel endless at the moment, they do shift and settle given proper care over time. We withdraw only to re-emerge stronger than imagined. Only by learning productive ways through the darkest moments can we develop skills and compassion that brightly light the way for others still struggling to find their way out of the depths in their own time too. There is hope for all.

Managing Emotions During Crises

When we find ourselves slammed by a crisis event, traumatic loss, or global disruption out of our control, the initial shock inevitably gives way to a flood of panic, sorrow, rage, anxiety, and despair. The sheer intensity of painful emotions in trauma's wake can seem relentless and endless. However using healthy coping strategies allows us to regain our footing while bearing unbearable pain skillfully, compassionately, and safely until the waves of distress naturally ease with time.

Identify Overwhelming Feelings

The first step in effectively managing powerful emotions following a crisis or tragedy involves simply identifying and labeling the feelings flooding our minds and bodies. Putting words to powerful sensations begins the process of moving pain from panicked places locked deep in nerve endings into thinking parts of the brain where we can better assess and address them. Is the emotion swirling within us abandonment, helplessness, anger, humiliation, regret, or fear? Labeling and acknowledging these emotions are half the battle.

Understand and Match Emotions

Next, actively work toward self-understanding around overwhelming emotions rather than harsh judgment or avoidance. Pain following tragedy is neither good nor bad—it just signals we are fully human with compassionate hearts that naturally break in response to undeserved suffering and injustice. Match the intensity and discomfort skillfully. Breathe with it, rock with it, scream with it, or cry with it. Fighting our natural flow only intensifies suffering. Flow with the waves skillfully instead.

Find Triggers

Carefully notice what external events or thoughts reliably seem to amplify painful inner states in the days following a crisis. Pinpointing these triggers creates awareness so we can better prepare to meet them with care and effective tools. Does interacting with certain personalities consistently produce anxiety? Do images of the traumatic event revive panic? Does visiting certain places create grief? Define vulnerabilities, then compassionately limit exposure or build emotional resources in advance to endure them.

Implement Coping Strategies

Once overwhelming sensations and reliable triggers are identified through non-judgmental understanding, we can then begin implementing targeted coping strategies, deliberately chosen to match and relieve each emotion.

For even more coping insights, visit the eighth chapter, exploring useful strategies such as emotional processing, establishing routines, and more. Tailor tools to fit the need. Handle anger with punching bags and restlessness with meditation, for example. And don't hesitate to ask guides for additional emotional management recommendations if you ever feel overwhelmed.

Seek Professional Help

In cases of sustained, unrelenting emotional turmoil following a crisis or loss, consult professional mental health support. Therapists, counselors, clergy, support groups, and crisis hotlines provide validating outside perspectives and teach research-backed skills for managing traumatic reactions. Tell others about uncontrolled thoughts of self-harm urgently. Help is ready when we're willing. You don't have to struggle alone.

Use Grounding Techniques

When painfully powerful feelings well up instantly, try grounding techniques to ease the intensity before implementing broader coping strategies. Find easy mental, physical, and soothing grounding skills to deploy at the moment when emotional waves crest and threaten to pull you under. Use apps with verbal cues. Caregivers can guide loved ones by naming grounding options out loud while the emotions pass.

By facing pain bravely through intense understanding and compassionately implementing skills that specifically match our unique inner space, we build emotional resilience while honoring the full humanity of our suffering. With consistent self-care and external support, we strengthen our capacity to skillfully bear even the unbearable—not perfectly or permanently, but just enough to keep walking forward when we want to collapse. In the process, we become living light whose hard-won wisdom brightens the way for other souls still struggling to push emotional boulders uphill alone. Take heart. Even this heaviness will pass.

Chapter 12:
The Long Game—Sustaining Resilience for Lifelong Well-being

How skillfully we navigate life's ups and downs determines the very quality of our existence. Yet most stumble through storms recklessly and ill-prepared, never pausing to actively strengthen emotional resilience before the next wave comes. Eventually, we grow so exhausted, dealing with crisis constantly, that we fall into depression, apathy, or defeat—believing our well-being an impossible ideal.

What if preventing prolonged suffering by wisely growing lasting, renewable resilience is the ultimate purpose that brings significance to our struggles? This last chapter helps you design your own customized resilience plan so that you can age with responsive flexibility, able to handle everyday stress as well as trauma.

Playing the long game means adopting a lifelong perspective with patience, realizing lasting behavioral change, and letting refined character emerge slowly from gathering wisdom along the journey. Quick fixes quickly dry out. But small, courageous steps build into lasting progress. Trusting the process allows us to release strict demands for immediate perfection, progression, or closure. We can rest in each precisely imperfect moment, neither overreacting to discomforts nor minimizing growth opportunities.

Patience also relieves us from judging progress by outcomes alone. Healing from painful ordeals depends on continually nurturing resilience despite the uncertainty ahead. Our primary scorecard for success becomes the honesty and compassion we bring to climbing life's hills today. Reward efforts now, not just distant goals that may remain forever out of distance. Celebrate small daily acts of stubborn grace.

The long game centers not on solving problems once and for all but on dancing with them as they come up, occasionally falling, and then recovering balance through careful adjustment to new environments and evolving emotional challenges. We don't resist pain as much as we skillfully welcome it as a teacher. Each storm makes us smarter guides, so those behind us gain smoother passage.

But even larger than the long game mindset is the infinite game perspective. While most play life as a game with a finale focused around one big goal, seeking to cross the finish triumphantly, infinite game players find purpose through continuing the journey itself with openness and abundance for all.

Infinite players thus lift not just themselves through struggle but guide others as comrades, releasing old hierarchical structures. They celebrate interdependence and teamwork, knowing winning rides upon communal resilience, not isolated victory through crushing opposition.

Therefore, the long game played well with open hands and radical inclusion, leads us into destinies far larger than ourselves alone. We become guides of a resilience legacy distributed equally by upholding the shared worth and strengths swimming in each soul. All we need to do is establish the conditions that help it surface.

So, shall we play? The infinite game awaits our first compassionate moves.

With a long-term perspective grounded firmly beneath us, we can begin practically building emotional resilience to last. We do this by specifically strengthening three key pillars continuously:

- **Self-reflection**: Regular reflection builds self-awareness, so we can catch unhealthy response patterns quickly without seeing them as permanent traits. Pause during adversity and ask, "What insights does this unpleasant emotion or limitation offer?" Uncover strengths rather than accepting damage as identity. Actively re-write limiting narratives over time by compassionately reinterpreting past pains as rich resources now.

- **Gratitude**: Nurturing daily gratitude for available supports, talents, and beauty softens trauma's sharp edges by balancing pain with acknowledged blessings. Gratitude lights hope. Regularly list specific appreciations and affirm thankfulness.

Even in dire lack or loss, air, sound, and sensations anchor us to basic goodness, from which we can slowly rebuild gratitude over time.

- **Self-compassion**: Silencing destructive inner critics also continues to foster resilience by nurturing emotional safety and warmth. Respond to insecurities with, "This feeling is hard. How might I gently care for myself in this state?" Imagine embracing struggling loved ones with unconditional compassion. Grant yourself an identical space.

Combined continually, they generate energy and flexibility, reaching through trauma now by soothing future selves who inherit this stored wisdom.

A practical metaphor for thinking of lifelong resilience practice involves visualizing our inner landscape as a garden, ripening toward abundant harvests only through skillful care. This garden is equally vulnerable to drought, weeds, erosion, overgrowth, or sudden storms. Purposeful resilience building thus becomes the ongoing work of attentive gardeners.

We actively tend to mental soil, turning yesterday's painful waste into tomorrow's fertile growth. We nurture relationships, providing protective barriers when harsh elements blow through. And we plant seeds of compassion, optimism, and purpose to give strength in the seasons ahead.

But neglect allows hard, weed-filled pathways of resentment, hostility, and perfectionism to stomp out individual wellness. So, we continually prune harmful thinking and beliefs that limit healthy responses. Storms test resilience, so we evaluate and strengthen the vulnerabilities in our mental infrastructure frequently. And when drought comes, we water weary parts with hope.

In these ways, through ongoing gardening, our inner acreage flourishes into resilient forests filled with fresh choices and contentment, accessible precisely when crises threaten to harm us. We're nourished by the lush spiritual ecosystem we've carefully grown well in advance—not despite struggles but through it.

Use the following prompts to begin practically building your personalized resilience plan with the long game in mind. Revisit them regularly to monitor progress and adapt strategies responsively over time as life circumstances and needs change.

- Take stock of current resilience levels across key dimensions—physical, social, emotional, professional, and spiritual. Which areas need strengthening most? Where are you already well supported?

- Recognize past situations that tested your resilience, successfully or unsuccessfully. Identify weak spots and common areas of vulnerability where focused skills training can better prepare you for next time.

- Who is part of your trusted supportive community, available to offer key resources as a backup when your resilience runs low? List names, strengths, and connections actively grown.

- What current self-care strategies effectively restore emotional balance and build highly flexible neural pathways through challenges? Which lifestyle factors exhaust our resilience? Detail a reasonable self-care regimen for this season, balancing competing priorities.

- Lastly, consider how actively developing resilience benefits you in ways other than your recovery. Imagine generational impacts as your strong branches become a safe place for others seeking space to strengthen roots within your empowering shade.

Along the way, crises will surely still arise. But their appearance becomes a reason for skillful engagement, not despair. With eyes towards the long game, we witness suffering shift while recognizing enduring wholeness underneath.

Through patient nurturing of insight, gratitude, and self-compassion across seasons, our motivation lasts longer against fear, anger, or shame. Thus strengthened collectively by the care we show ourselves and those beside us now, no storm needs to sweep us all away ever again. We shine too brightly, and we love too boldly. The long game makes us infinite.

Onward now with care, courage, and joy toward the horizon, always magnificently unfolding ahead. This vision still grows.

Perseverance Prevails: The Importance of Ongoing Resilience Nurturing

Bouncing back from adversity requires more than waiting passively for challenges to pass and wounds to close in due time. True resilience emerges through action and perspective shifts that actively transform crises into opportunities for growth, from which we bloom stronger, wiser, and more compassionate. It is our tireless nurturing through storms that allows us to rise above destructive waves threatening to overwhelm us. We endure the unendurable by soothing our inner landscapes skillfully, not avoiding external pains.

The Power of Perseverance

Resilience, at its core, means persevering despite hardship and uncertainty. It is stubborn, willful choosing of potential over pain day after day until tiny victories build up suddenly into courage and expanded ability we hardly recognize.

Like determined drops cutting mighty canyons through stone slowly, we focus not on the size of obstacles before us but on the daily pressure we apply, with a commitment to making our way through despite whatever comes our way. In this way, perseverance proves itself to be the bedrock of every achievement and the DNA of dreams, especially resilience.

Resilience Nature's Way

Consider how a forest ecosystem offers a meaningful metaphor for understanding true resilience. Trees don't just wait idly, hoping lightning strikes will spare them. They actively adapt to even devastating fires, floods, and viruses by putting out shoots, seasoning bark beyond burning, and sending roots deeper into new soil.

In the same way, we must consistently choose growth, repeatedly following life's inevitable heartbreaks and traumas until productive responses outpace doubt, despair, and destruction. With perseverant effort, we gradually transform fiery trials into nutrients, nourishing fruits of insight and maturity over time. Survival alone gives way to redemption only through persistent nurturing, despite adversity.

Cultivating Continuity

Unlike support that comes in only after a crisis, authentic resilience building requires continuity through organizations proactively providing supportive resources, processes, and mindsets into cultural infrastructure before disasters strike.

For example, continuity planning builds organizational resilience by addressing threats, defining important functions, preparing leadership, and cross-training staff as failure backup. Testing plans frequently then strengthens responsiveness. Industries that simply react prove far more vulnerable to struggles than those grounding operations in carefully constructed foundations that survive despite disruption.

The very essence of building durable resilience whether personal or communal, depends upon persistently nurturing contributive factors continuously over time. This must be done until they grow roots strong enough to withstand unpredictable storms and carry communities through to thriving stability on the other side. Only perseverant initiative beats back adversity's threats.

Long-Term Benefits of Resilience Nurturing

Cultivating personal and collective resilience before crises strike requires heroic measures that not only equip us to endure immediate troubles but also build up payoffs that help us through lifetimes and generations beyond. The long game builds up more and more over time. Consider how dedication to nurturing resilience produces these far-reaching benefits:

- **Sustainable and inclusive growth**: Economies and organizations built upon inclusive, diverse contributions and sustainable practices grow resilient to market uncertainties. They allow broader inputs and distribute backup. They survive downturns readily and bounce back stronger, serving wider stakeholders in the long term.

- **Adaptability**: Regular disruption creates innovation as groups adapt to welcome changing realities. Resilience focuses less on protecting old ways and more on welcoming new possibilities and combinations unlocked by crises. Change builds capacity.

- **Cost savings**: Resilience lowers healthcare costs by nurturing employee well-being and organizational stability. Turnover, insurance premiums, and missed days decline dramatically when populations develop the skills to endure adversity in the workplace and in life.

- **Improved mental health**: Deliberately honing cognitive, emotional, and communal supports before trauma reduces the rate of prolonged PTSD symptoms, clinical anxiety, and depression. Proactive resilience building prevents issues from building up over time.

- **Competitive advantage**: Organizational resilience is the ultimate competitive advantage in modern global uncertainty. No single crisis can easily damage adaptive systems with distributed resources to access in times of struggle.

- **Improved organizational health**: Strengthening operational resilience ahead of any crisis boosts critical communication loops, succession strategies, diversity, and supply chain flexibility to reduce business disruption. What survives builds fitness.

- **Increased stability**: Individuals and groups who learn to navigate troubles without lasting catastrophic damage create shields of institutional wisdom and stability, uplifting community morale, productivity, and innovation in the long term.

- **Enhanced social and environmental practices**: Crafting organizational resilience around inclusive environmental, social, and governance priorities with ethical supply chains and accountability measures bakes responsiveness into corporate culture, uplifting society broadly.

- **Lifelong journey of renewal**: While formal training can provide initial crisis response skills and trauma healing tools, crafting resilience across a lifespan depends fundamentally upon continuously choosing small acts of renewal through adversity. With practice and persistence, facing troubles and uncertainty little by little with whatever scrappy resources we have at the moment, we gradually build endurance for even greater trials ahead.

Over decades, these perseverant choices build up into vast resilience without bounds. Until one day we realize a wellspring of wisdom and grace ever deepening at our core—collective waters gathering streams of hardship, endured so skillfully that no tragedy, however immense, can ever weaken the watershed.

Here wells resilience eternal. We prevail at last.

Building Resilience Practices

In our fast-paced, connected yet disconnected modern age, actively building emotional resilience serves as essential armor, protecting well-being from stress. Without prevention strategies to ease impacts, we risk rapid physical and mental decline. Use the proven tips below to design your tailored proactive resilience action plan.

Be sure to incorporate supportive self-care habits from Chapter 7 as well, like consistent healthy nutrition, sufficient sleep and rest, regular exercise, and stress management rhythms. Tiny daily wellness practices build up over decades into powerful lifelong fitness.

Get Connected

Humans thrive on shared experience and connection. Yet many neglect nourishing important supportive connections that provide outlets for processing adversity and accountability through struggles. Identify and regularly engage both close intimate circles and broader communities aligning values with your own as touchstones when you need reassurance, perspective, or assistance. Especially in crises, isolation increases hopelessness. Stay plugged in.

Learn From the Past and Develop a Sense of Purpose

Reflect often on formative episodes from your past, especially difficult ones, to find constructive themes that reveal core strengths grown through your story. Identify how every phase has prepared you uniquely for now. Understanding the development of inner grit already demonstrated builds confidence to rely on that resilience again when you need it next.

Furthermore, claim authorship of your narrative without shame or self-pity. Responsibly acknowledge past contributions without blaming outside forces for lasting harm or defining identity through tragedy forever. Our narratives become the very backbone supporting overall wellness and purpose.

Find Meaning in Every Day

Seek significance through consistency in small deeds, not hungering after big breaks. Show up with your presence for the simple joys and responsibilities already gracing today. Fulfillment hides in plain sight when we exist in our twenty-four hours consciously, embracing the now.

Refuel and Stay Hopeful

Prioritize activities reliably, boosting your optimism, creativity, and motivation. Refuel yourself through uplifting music, comedy, inspirational reading, nature, and play. Stay immersed in hopeful media, avoiding excessive exposure to negative reports that only make you feel helpless. Actively nourish positive emotional states so you have strength when adversity strikes without warning.

Practice Thought Awareness

Like doing reps in the gym builds muscular strength, exercising conscious power over thoughts develops mental fitness by turning experiences into growth. Replace unrealistic thinking with balanced perspectives. Redirect harmful self-criticisms into compassion and encouragement. Allow emotions without overreacting to their implications. Developing thought awareness builds resilience to roll with life's ups and downs with less suffering.

Take Care of Yourself

Monitor energy spent closely across key dimensions—emotional, physical, financial, and mental—and budget it deliberately to save margins in preparation for sudden trouble. Set healthy boundaries around work, social media, and worrying about events beyond your control. Decrease needless stress by finding the space and adequate rest required for developing resilience. Allow yourself to protect your sanity first. The long-term strategy depends on you wisely identifying the drain from essential priorities for sustainable thriving.

Take Action and Identify Priorities

Resilience emerges only through repeated exposure, developing attitudes and behaviors slowly against destructive thinking in action. So, purposefully welcome constructive discomfort by acting courageously on behalf of growth, even when feeling fearful or unprepared. State intentions, identify top priorities amid competing demands, then structure habits, steadily building emotional and situational management skills through accountability. Progress rewards action.

Adopt a Positive Perspective

In every circumstance, consciously choose to resolve to find benefits from the situation rather than thinking endlessly about the problem itself. Ask empowering questions like, "What hidden gifts emerge here?" or "How can this strengthen me?" That pivot toward learning through challenges ultimately drives positive transformation out of suffering. Reframing experiences constructively builds resilience automatically.

Take Personal Responsibility

While validating external traumatic causes, also own your power to respond or react to events positively. Blaming outside forces only for prolonged troubles or emotional disruption hands away your agency. Aim for anger appropriately, then proactively accept imperfect scenarios as the very building blocks setting up your growth. Through facing down pain and committing to learning from the experience, we prepare ourselves to deal with the next situation in an even better way.

By incorporating such resilience-boosting practices into our daily lifestyle, we strengthen mental muscles and neural pathways, slowly allowing us to overcome mountains of adversity. Built up over the years, small, courageous, constructive choices have become the very foundation for upholding unconditional well-being. No one incident can shake us ever again. We bloom perennials despite crushing winter storms by wisely utilizing each season in turn to strengthen deeper roots next time—transformed through the very trials we once believed would destroy us. Now we mightily prevail.

Reflection, Gratitude, Compassion—The Trio of Sustained Resilience

Cultivating deep, lifelong resilience depends less on perfecting reactions in isolated moments of adversity and more on continually nurturing three essential skills: self-reflection, gratitude practice, and self-compassion.

Together, they instill a perspective that is immediately accessible precisely when traumatic pain or despair threatens to overcome our coping capacity completely. Mastering this trio develops profound balance, whatever external chaos swirls.

The Role of Self-Reflection

Turning attention inward regularly builds awareness of subconscious patterns otherwise triggered unexpectedly, sending us into fight, flight, or freeze. By continually monitoring thought processes and emotions flowing beneath the surface as we move through daily events, sudden flare-ups hold fewer surprises that might overwhelm us in a crisis.

We can name and compassionately work with intense anger when internal red flags go up instead of lashing out regrettably. We catch ourselves before diving down mental rabbit holes. We shift gears the instant we recognize our thoughts spinning unproductively.

This self-attunement muscle develops instincts for catching limiting narratives before they happen by routinely testing thoughts objectively against the core truths we know rationally. "Do recurring self-attacks accurately represent my character?" "Is this anxiety exaggerated beyond current facts?" Such introspection creates internal stability.

Furthermore, the self-knowledge gained through routine reflection allows us to design targeted practices addressing areas of vulnerability or dysfunction. This allows us to have them ready in times of crisis, exactly when we need inner support the most to stay afloat through external storms.

At important times, perceived victimization gives way to self-empowerment when we look inward and discover areas we can improve instead. The difference between sinking and swimming often pivots here upon this compassionate sight, granting vision to heal—or at least endure—brutal seas churning within and without.

Thus, self-reflection sustains resilience as we uncover, then lovingly convert emotional baggage into gold, remove unrealistic ideas of our reality, and then navigate confidently despite the oppressive fog. The self-aware walk back upright, however long the uncertain roads ahead may be. Inside, we glow brightly.

The Power of Gratitude

Like athletes cross-training muscle groups to balance overall fitness, shifting mental focus toward blessing oneself counters trauma's damage when we focus entirely on painful losses or injustice experienced. Counting our gifts in the aftermath builds much-needed perspective.

By naming specifics we remain grateful for even amid struggles, we limit the panic trauma wields, showing us the glimmers of goodness unable to be fully removed. This act of radical gratefulness grounds us in a direct sensory experience at the moment. We realize beauty, order, and pleasure are still available at this very moment if we pause to access them.

Gratitude grants us eyes to finally recognize what we still have, the things hidden away when our tears blind us to them. When we actively participate in regular thankful thoughts, neural pathways wire themselves towards abundance versus lack, no matter how little we have left after a loss. Our whole perception shifts from loss to wholeness, still subtly helping us rebuild.

Over weeks and years, as focusing on thankfulness grows habitual, we grow the capacity to find the good in any struggle thus resiliently turning misfortune into unexpected triumph. By keeping up our spirit through gratitude, we not only learn to persist through hard times but grow stronger as a result of them.

Cultivating Self-Compassion

Critical to maintaining resilience long-term, self-compassion involves learning to actively comfort ourselves with warmth when distress feels unrelenting. This means first silencing toxic inner voices and stopping the habit of instantly blaming, shaming or panicking around struggles. Breathe through the trouble, directing attention back to facts, not exaggerated stories created in moments of anxiety. Release judgments that failure determines your self-worth. Fighting made-up demons further exhausts energy reserves already exhausted in the crisis.

Transition instead with gentle understanding for the suffering that all well-intentioned souls stumble into at times. Talk respectfully with yourself, as you would a beloved friend dealing with harsh circumstances.

"This difficult season is more than I can handle right now, but I trust a solution will appear." Hug the parts of you that are hurting. Encourage yourself audibly.

Core to this process is accepting fallibility and confusion as normal aspects of lifelong growth. Expect setbacks to arise and celebrate small daily courage despite imperfection. Scan your memory for previous hard times that were navigated successfully, and learn from them. Validate your strength and past skills in overcoming adversity, even if outcomes now seem uncertain or it feels like you don't have the strength to cope. Storms pass. Resilience flows as we support self-talk with unyielding compassion, building sufficient love within to outlast the storms ahead. Defenseless no more, we patiently reinforce this self-love until the fields between us and the violent world bloom lush and bright.

Thus, ongoing self-care brings in eventual redemption where trauma first hammered cruelly. Wounds transform into wisdom, one sustained act of grace at a time, till glory arrives.

We journey home this way. May compassion light long roads before you until your arrival, where anguish ends and joy unwavering rises gentle but firm as dawn's first light, healing hurt held beyond the too-long night of the soul. Once broken hearts mend, they can mend again.

Conclusion

As we reach the end of our resilience journey together, I hope that you feel empowered by the knowledge and practical strategies shared within these pages. Whether you picked up this book out of personal interest or professional necessity, my goal was to provide an accessible guide to understanding, nurturing, and sustaining our remarkable human capacity to bounce back from adversity.

Resilience remains one of the most crucial abilities we can grow to thrive in an increasingly complex world. The many personal stories of resilience triumphing over tragedy, the science illuminating resilience's foundations, and the diverse practical techniques for strengthening resilience all testify to the incredible potential within us all to transform challenges into growth.

While each chapter covered specific dimensions of resilience—from the biological to the social to the emotional realms—a key lesson woven throughout is that resilience does not exist in isolation. Like an intricate web, the many strands of our lives interconnect to determine how we respond to hardship. Resilience relies on the body and brain working in harmony, the heart and mind aligned, and our interpersonal bonds providing ballast through life's storms.

The multidimensional nature of resilience highlights why diverse evidence-based strategies prove vital. Whether honing communication skills for seeking social support, practicing mindfulness to manage stress, or adopting self-care habits that nurture overall well-being, small, consistent actions cultivate the built-up interest in resilience over time. Momentum builds, neural pathways are wired, and social safety nets are woven tighter.

Yet the private intensity of inner resilience-building work cannot be underestimated. From discovering motivation through soul-searching self-reflection to confronting disempowering assumptions that hijack potential, the inside job of resilience asks much of us. It demands brutal honesty, courageous self-awareness, and the humility to accept our essential fallibility.

However, the personal potential restored through this tough work allows us to spread the ripples of resilience ever wider. Because resilient people lead resilient families, resilient families build resilient communities, and so on. Each small act of resilience-building therefore holds revolutionary potential for positive transformation.

As the final chapter's title suggests, resilience is truly a lifelong journey with occasional milestones rather than a finite destination. Our work is never complete. Challenges will continue arising, assumptions need revisiting, and skills are always improving. But with a factual understanding of resilience now yours and evidence-based techniques in your toolkit, you hold the power to take responsibility for building your resilience muscle often, bit by bit.

My parting advice is to be gentle with yourself but maintain a consistent awareness of nurturing your resilience. Journal occasional check-ins to audit your resilience health—are you sleeping enough? Have you connected meaningfully with loved ones recently? Are you staying active? If you notice your resilience battery running low, act swiftly to implement a "resilience pit stop" through restorative self-care.

I also encourage you to pay the lessons forward by shining the light left by your resilience during times of darkness. Seek opportunities big and small to role model resilience habits, share techniques with others who are struggling, or simply radiate resilient energy through random acts of kindness. Building community resilience amplifies our individual bounce-back capacity exponentially.

As your partner along this path of discovery and growth, I sincerely hope reading this book left you feeling more inspired, informed, and empowered to unleash your inner capacities for resilience. May you face all future storms with courage, stand tall through the turbulence, and ultimately bounce ever forward into positive possibility. Our greatest glory as humans lies not in never falling but in rising every time we fall. Remember, life does not throw you stones; it gives you building blocks.

Glossary

- **Acceptance:** Willingness to tolerate difficult situations without attempting to change them.

- **Adaptability:** Ability to adjust to new conditions.

- **Adversity:** Difficult situations and hardships in life.

- **Balance:** Harmony is created by adjusting different elements appropriately.

- **Bounce-back:** The ability to recover quickly from setbacks.

- **Bravery:** The quality of facing pain or danger with determination and confidence.

- **Burnout:** Physical or mental collapse due to overwork or stress.

- **Commitment:** Dedication to keep applying effort toward a challenging goal.

- **Compassion:** Sympathy for the suffering of others.

- **Coping:** Dealing effectively with a difficult situation.

- **Crisis:** A time of intense difficulty or danger.

- **Emotions:** Natural instinctive feelings derived from one's circumstances.

- **Empowerment:** Authority or power given to someone to do something.

- **Fortitude:** Strength of mind that allows facing adversity with bravery.

- **Fulfillment:** A sense of purpose, meaning, and satisfaction in life.

- **Gratitude:** Appreciation and thankfulness for what one has.

- **Grit:** Passionate perseverance toward long-term goals despite obstacles.

- **Hardship:** Severe suffering or deprivation.

- **Insight:** Deep understanding that helps make positive change.

- **Integrity:** The quality of being honest and having strong morals and principles.

- **Mindfulness:** Focusing one's awareness on the present moment.

- **Presence:** The focus of one's conscious attention in the current moment.

- **Perseverance:** Persistence in doing something despite difficulty.

- **Purpose:** The reason for which something is done or created.

- **Reflection:** A serious thought or consideration.

- **Resilience:** The capacity to recover quickly from difficulties.

- **Resolute:** Admirably purposeful, determined, and unwavering.

- **Responsibility:** Being accountable for one's actions.

- **Self-awareness:** Conscious knowledge of one's character and feelings.

- **Tenacity:** Persistence in sticking to decisions and courses of action.

- **Transformation:** A marked change in nature or appearance.

- **Wisdom:** Knowledge and experience needed to make sensible decisions.

References

Abrams, Z. (2022, October 1). *Student mental health is in crisis. Campuses are rethinking their approach.* American Psychological Association. https://www.apa.org/monitor/2022/10/mental-health-campus-care

Akers, A. S. (2023, August 3). *Preventing burnout: 7 strategies and when to seek help.* MedicalNewsToday. https://www.medicalnewstoday.com/articles/preventing-burnout

Arida, R. M., & Teixeira-Machado, L. (2021). The Contribution of Physical Exercise to Brain Resilience. *Frontiers in Behavioral Neuroscience, 14*(20). https://doi.org/10.3389/fnbeh.2020.626769

Baldoni, J. (2017, December 13). *5 Inspirational Stories of Resilience.* Forbes. https://www.forbes.com/sites/johnbaldoni/2017/12/13/5-inspirational-stories-of-resilience/?sh=44e37e7b426b

Booth, J. (2023, October 19). *Anxiety Statistics and Facts.* Forbes Health. https://www.forbes.com/health/mind/anxiety-statistics/

Bravely Team (2022, March 29). *The biggest myths about resilience in the workplace.* Bravely. https://workbravely.com/blog/culture-transformation/the-biggest-myths-about-resilience-at-work/

Cathomas, F., Murrough, J. W., Nestler, E. J., Han, M.-H., & Russo, S. J. (2019). Neurobiology of resilience: Interface between mind and body. *Biological Psychiatry, 86*(6). https://doi.org/10.1016/j.biopsych.2019.04.011

Centers for Disease Control and Prevention. (2019, May 1). *Anxiety and depression in children: Get the facts.*

https://www.cdc.gov/childrensmentalhealth/features/anxiety-depression-children.html

Chan, C. K. Y. (2021). *Resilience.* Holistic Competency & Virtue Education. https://www.have.hku.hk/resilience

Chan, K. (2023, June 16). *5 Types of Adversity and Ways to Overcome Them.* Verywell Mind. https://www.verywellmind.com/types-of-adversity-and-ways-to-overcome-them-7505840

Cherry, K. (2022, February 23). *Why Communication In Relationships Is So Important.* Verywell Mind. https://www.verywellmind.com/communication-in-relationships-why-it-matters-and-how-to-improve-5218269

Cherry, K. (2023, March 15). *What is Resilience?* Verywell Mind. https://www.verywellmind.com/characteristics-of-resilience-2795062

Cherry, K. (2023, May 3). *How Resilience Helps You Cope With Life's Challenges.* Verywell Mind. https://www.verywellmind.com/what-is-resilience-2795059

Clark, M. (2021, August 19). *50+ Shocking Physician Burnout Statistics You'll Never Believe.* Etactics. https://etactics.com/blog/physician-burnout-statistics

Cohn, M. A., Fredrickson, B. L., Brown, S. L., Mikels, J. A., & Conway, A. M. (2009). Happiness unpacked: Positive emotions increase life satisfaction by building resilience. *Emotion, 9*(3), 361–368. https://doi.org/10.1037/a0015952

Collado-Soler, R., Trigueros, R., Aguilar-Parra, J. M., & Navarro, N. (2023). Emotional Intelligence and Resilience Outcomes in Adolescent Period, is Knowledge Really Strength? *Psychology Research and Behavior Management, 2023*(16), 1365–1378. https://doi.org/10.2147/prbm.s383296

Craig, H. (2019, January 16). *Resilience in the Workplace: How to Be Resilient at Work.* PositivePsychology. https://positivepsychology.com/resilience-in-the-workplace/

Cuffari, B. (2023, April 11). *Does Loneliness Weaken the Immune System?* News Medical. https://www.news-medical.net/health/Does-Loneliness-Weaken-the-Immune-System.aspx

Cullins, A. (2021, July 9). *Fixed Mindset vs. Growth Mindset Examples.* Big Life Journal. https://biglifejournal.com/blogs/blog/fixed-mindset-vs-growth-mindset-examples

Davis, P. (2016, February 8). *5 Myths About Resilience.* Forbes. https://www.forbes.com/sites/pauladavislaack/2016/02/08/5-myths-about-resilience/

Dhungana, S., Koirala, R., Ojha, S. P., & Thapa, S. B. (2022). Resilience and its association with post-traumatic stress disorder, anxiety, and depression symptoms in the aftermath of trauma: A cross-sectional study from Nepal. *SSM - Mental Health, 2,* 100135. https://doi.org/10.1016/j.ssmmh.2022.100135

Dziurkowska, E., & Wesolowski, M. (2021). Cortisol as a Biomarker of Mental Disorder Severity. *Journal of Clinical Medicine, 10*(21), 5204. https://doi.org/10.3390/jcm10215204

Ellwood-Lowe, M. E., Irving, C. N., & Bunge, S. A. (2022). Exploring neural correlates of behavioral and academic resilience among children in poverty. *Developmental Cognitive Neuroscience, 54,* 101090. https://doi.org/10.1016/j.dcn.2022.101090

Fleming, J., & Ledogar, R. J. (2018). Resilience, an Evolving Concept: A Review of Literature Relevant to Aboriginal Research. *Pimatisiwin, 6*(2), 7–23. https://www.ncbi.nlm.nih.gov/pmc/articles/PMC2956753/

Fowler, P. (2018, January 11). *Breathing Techniques for Stress Relief.* WebMD. https://www.webmd.com/balance/stress-management/stress-relief-breathing-techniques

Garcia, A. C. M., Ferreira, A. C. G., Silva, L. S. R., da Conceição, V. M., Nogueira, D. A., & Mills, J. (2022). Mindful Self-Care, Self-Compassion, and Resilience Among Palliative Care Providers During the COVID-19 Pandemic. *Journal of Pain and Symptom*

Management, *64*(1). https://doi.org/10.1016/j.jpainsymman.2022.03.003

Harvard College. (2019, May 14). *An active social life may help you live longer.* https://www.hsph.harvard.edu/news/hsph-in-the-news/active-social-life-longevity/

Hemphill, B. E. (2022, December 6). *Uncomfortable (but Necessary) Conversations About Burnout.* Gallup. https://www.gallup.com/workplace/406232/uncomfortable-necessary-conversations-burnout.aspx

Hetherington, C. (2023, November 11). *The Power of Social Connection for Longevity.* HealthNews. https://healthnews.com/longevity/healthspan/social-connection-and-longevity/

Hurley, K. (2019, December 14). *A Guide to Facing Life's Challenges and Adversities.* Castle Connolly. https://www.castleconnolly.com/topics/self-nurturing/guide-to-resilience

Idris, I., Khairani, A. Z., & Shamsuddin, H. (2019). The Influence of Resilience on Psychological Well-Being of Malaysian University Undergraduates. *International Journal of Higher Education, 8*(4), 153. https://doi.org/10.5430/ijhe.v8n4p153

Israelashvili, J. (2021). More Positive Emotions During the COVID-19 Pandemic are Associated With Better Resilience, Especially for Those Experiencing More Negative Emotions. *Frontiers in Psychology, 12.* https://doi.org/10.3389/fpsyg.2021.648112

Janitra, F. E., Jen, H.-J., Chu, H., Chen, R., Pien, L.-C., Liu, D., Lai, Y.-J., Banda, K. J., Lee, T.-Y., Lin, H.-C., Chang, C.-Y., & Chou, K.-R. (2023). Global prevalence of low resilience among the general population and health professionals during the COVID-19 pandemic: A meta-analysis. *Journal of Affective Disorders, 332,* 29–46. https://doi.org/10.1016/j.jad.2023.03.077

Karunyam, B. V., Karim, A., Mohamed, I. N., Ugusman, A., Mohamed, W., Ahmad, M., Abu, M. A., & Kumar, J. (2023). Infertility and cortisol: A systematic review. *Frontiers in Endocrinology, 14.* https://doi.org/10.3389/fendo.2023.1147306

Kontoangelos, K., Raptis, A., Lambadiari, V., Economou, M., Tsiori, S., Katsi, V., Papageorgiou, C., Martinaki, S., Dimitriadis, G., & Papageorgiou, C. (2022). Burnout Related to Diabetes Mellitus: A Critical Analysis. *Clinical Practice and Epidemiology in Mental Health, 18*(1). https://doi.org/10.2174/17450179-v18-e2209010

Koutsimani, P., Montgomery, A., & Georganta, K. (2019). The Relationship Between Burnout, Depression, and Anxiety: A Systematic Review and Meta-Analysis. *Frontiers in Psychology, 10*(284). https://doi.org/10.3389/fpsyg.2019.00284

Kushwaha, Y., Chakravarty, T. R., & Srivastava, A. (2022). A Study on Happiness and Resilience with the Reference to the Professional Students of Higher Education: A Thematical Analysis. *YMER, 21(12),* 672-682. https://ymerdigital.com/uploads/YMER2112B6.pdf

Li, P. (2020, August 1). *Resilience Theory in Psychology (Definition & Characteristics).* Parenting for Brain. https://www.parentingforbrain.com/resilience-theory/

Linder, N., Giusti, M., Samuelsson, K., & Barthel, S. (2021). Pro-environmental habits: An underexplored research agenda in sustainability science. *Ambio: A Journal of Environment and Society, 51,* 546-556. https://doi.org/10.1007/s13280-021-01619-6

Marriage.com Editorial Team. (2021, June 23). *The importance of communication in relationships.* Marriage.com. https://www.marriage.com/advice/communication/importance-of-communication-in-relationships/

Maul, S., Giegling, I., Fabbri, C., Corponi, F., Serretti, A., & Rujescu, D. (2019). Genetics of resilience: Implications from genome-wide association studies and candidate genes of the stress response system in posttraumatic stress disorder and depression. *American*

Journal of Medical Genetics Part B: Neuropsychiatric Genetics, 183(2). https://doi.org/10.1002/ajmg.b.32763

McEwen, B. S. (2019, January 1). Chapter 2 - Resilience of the Brain and Body. *Stress: Physiology, Biochemistry, and Pathology, 3*. https://www.sciencedirect.com/science/article/abs/pii/B9780128131466000023

Melkonian, L. (2021, February 11). *What is emotional well-being? 8 ways to improve your mental health*. BetterUp. https://www.betterup.com/blog/what-is-emotional-well-being

Moodfit Staff. (2021, October 6). *Habits & Mental Health: The Importance of Building Resilience*. Moodfit. https://www.getmoodfit.com/post/habits-mental-health-the-importance-of-building-resilience

Navrady, L. B., Zeng, Y., Clarke, T.-K., Adams, M. J., Howard, D. M., Deary, I. J., & McIntosh, A. M. (2018). Genetic and environmental contributions to psychological resilience and coping. *Wellcome Open Research, 3*, 12. https://doi.org/10.12688/wellcomeopenres.13854.1

O'Neill, E. (2021, August 16). *10 Strategies For Managing Emotions*. Langley Group. https://langleygroup.com.au/10-strategies-for-managing-emotions/

Oestreicher, C. (2007). A history of chaos theory. *Dialogues in Clinical Neuroscience, 9*(3), 279–289. https://www.ncbi.nlm.nih.gov/pmc/articles/PMC3202497/

Parmar, R. (2022, May 10). *The Science of Resilience and Wisdom*. The University of Chicago. https://wisdomcenter.uchicago.edu/news/wisdom-news/science-resilience-and-wisdom

Ravitz, A. (2023, November 6). *How to Foster Resilience in Kids*. Child Mind Institute. https://childmind.org/article/foster-resilience-kids/

Rege, S. (2020, April 4). *Neurobiology of Stress and Resilience*. Psych Scene Hub. https://psychscenehub.com/psychinsights/neurobiology-of-stress-and-resilience/

Ristevska-Dimitrovska, G., Filov, I., Rajchanovska, D., Stefanovski, P., & Dejanova, B. (2015). Resilience and Quality of Life in Breast Cancer Patients. *Open Access Macedonian Journal of Medical Sciences*, *3*(4), 727–731. https://doi.org/10.3889/oamjms.2015.128

Salzberg, S. (2018, June 6). *RAIN: A mindfulness practice for welcoming your emotions*. Mindful. https://www.mindful.org/rain-a-mindfulness-practice-for-welcoming-your-emotions/

Saxler, P. K., Luk, G., Harris, P., & Gabrieli, J. (2016). *The Marshmallow Test: Delay of Gratification and Independent Rule Compliance*. https://dash.harvard.edu/bitstream/handle/1/27112705/SAXLER-DISSERTATION-2016.pdf?sequence=1&isAllowed=y

Sutton, J. (2019, January 3). *What is Resilience and why is it Important to Bounce Back?* PositivePsychology. https://positivepsychology.com/what-is-resilience/

Swaminathan, A., Gliksberg, M., Anbalagan, S., Wigoda, N., & Levkowitz, G. (2023). Stress resilience is established during development and is regulated by complement factors. *Cell Reports*, *42*(1), 111973. https://doi.org/10.1016/j.celrep.2022.111973

Tabibnia, G., & Radecki, D. (2018). Resilience training that can change the brain. *Consulting Psychology Journal: Practice and Research*, *70*(1), 59–88. https://doi.org/10.1037/cpb0000110

Talarico, J. N. de S., Marin, M.-F., Sindi, S., & Lupien, S. J. (2011). Effects of stress hormones on the brain and cognition: Evidence from normal to pathological aging. *Dementia & Neuropsychologia*, *5*(1), 8–16. https://doi.org/10.1590/s1980-57642011dn05010003

Tugade, M. M., & Fredrickson, B. L. (2004). Resilient individuals use positive emotions to bounce back from negative emotional experiences. *Journal of Personality and Social Psychology, 86*(2), 320–333. https://doi.org/10.1037/0022-3514.86.2.320

Wang, Z., Whiteside, S., Sim, L., Farah, W., Morrow, A., Alsawas, M., Moreno, P. B., Tello, M., Asi, N., Beuschel, B., Daraz, L., Almasri, J., Zaiem, F., Gunjal, S., Mantilla, L. L., Ponte, O. P., LeBlanc, A., Prokop, L. J., & Murad, M. H. (2017). Anxiety in children. In *www.ncbi.nlm.nih.gov*. Agency for Healthcare Research and Quality (US). https://www.ncbi.nlm.nih.gov/books/NBK476265/

World Health Organization. (2022, March 2). *COVID-19 pandemic triggers 25% increase in prevalence of anxiety and depression worldwide.* https://www.who.int/news/item/02-03-2022-covid-19-pandemic-triggers-25-increase-in-prevalence-of-anxiety-and-depression-worldwide

Yang, C., Zhou, Y., Cao, Q., Xia, M., & An, J. (2019). The Relationship Between Self-Control and Self-Efficacy Among Patients With Substance use Disorders: Resilience and self-esteem as mediators. *Frontiers in Psychiatry, 10.* https://doi.org/10.3389/fpsyt.2019.00388

www.ingramcontent.com/pod-product-compliance
Lightning Source LLC
Chambersburg PA
CBHW010448010526
44118CB00019B/2509